ABOUT THE AUTHOR

Maryon Stewart studied preventive dentistry and nutrition at the Royal Dental Hospital in London and worked as a counsellor with nutritional doctors in England for four years. At the beginning of 1984 she set up the PMT Advisory Service which has subsequently helped thousands of women world-wide. In 1987 she launched the Women's Nutritional Advisory Service which now provides broader help to women of all ages, all over the world.

Maryon Stewart is the author of the best-selling books *Beat the Menopause Without HRT*, *No More PMS*, *Beat Sugar Craving*, *Healthy Parents, Healthy Baby*, *The Zest for Life Plan* and a new book *Cruising Through the Menopause*. She is also the co-author of *No More IBS*, *Beat PMS Cookbook* and *Every Woman's Health Guide*. She has her own weekly radio programme on health and nutrition, has co-written several medical papers and has written for many glossy magazines and for the national daily newspapers.

She has appeared on many TV programmes on all five channels, has had regular pages in *House and Garden*, *Healthy Eating* and *Good Health* magazines and is on the Expert Panel for *Top Santé* magazine. She now writes regularly for *The Sunday Express Magazine* and was voted one of the most influential women in Great Britain in a *Good Housekeeping* Survey. She frequently lectures to both the public and medical profession. She is married to Dr Alan Stewart; they live in Lewes, Sussex, with their four children.

*Nor love, nor honour, wealth nor pow'r, can give the
heart a cheerful hour when health is lost.*

Be timely wise; with health all taste of pleasure flies.

John Gray, 'Ode on Vicissitude' 1.95.

Other titles by Maryon Stewart

No More PMS!
No More IBS!
Cruising Through the Menopause
Beat Sugar Craving
Healthy Parents, Healthy Baby
Every Woman's Health Guide
Maryon Stewart's Zest for Life Plan

THE PHYTO
FACTOR

*A revolutionary way to boost overall health
– reducing the risk of cancer, heart disease
and osteoporosis – and to control the
menopause naturally*

Maryon Stewart

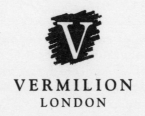

VERMILION
LONDON

To Alan – you are the 'wind beneath my wings'

1 3 5 7 9 10 8 6 4 2

Text copyright © Maryon Stewart 1998, 2000

Maryon Stewart has asserted her right to be identified as the author of
this work under the Copyright, Designs and Patents Act 1988.

First published in the United Kingdom in 1998 by Vermilion
This new edition first publishing in the United Kingdom in 2000
by Vermilion an imprint of Ebury Press
Random House
20 Vauxhall Bridge Road
London SW1V 2SA

Random House South Africa (Pty) Limited
Endulini, 5A Jubilee Road,
Parktown 2193, South Africa

The Random House Group Limited Reg. No. 954009

www.randomhouse.co.uk

A CIP catalogue record for this book is available from the
British Library

ISBN: 0 09 185655 8

Papers used by Vermilion are natural, recyclable products made from
wood grown in sustainable forests.

Printed and bound in Great Britain by Mackays of Chatham plc,
Chatham, Kent

Although every effort has been made to ensure that the
contents of this book are accurate, it must not be treated as a substitute for qualified medical advice. Always
consult a qualified medical practitioner. Neither the
Author nor the Publisher can be held responsible for
any loss or claim arising out of the use, or misuse, of the
suggestions made or the failure to take medical advice.

CONTENTS

ACKNOWLEDGEMENTS

Writing a book is never easy for me as I have a full-time occupation looking after the Women's Nutritional Advisory Service (WNAS) and a family of four children. In order to get words on the page I usually have to creep off somewhere peaceful, clutching my word processor. This time was no exception, but for one factor. There were so many research papers to read I couldn't carry them, but instead had to have them delivered in a huge parcel. Therefore, my first thanks must go to the many scientists and researchers around the world who have opened my eyes to a discovery which is likely to dramatically improve our health prospects. Professor Herman Adlercreutz, from the Department of Clinical Chemistry at the University of Helsinki should be first on the list, since he has undoubtedly engineered so much of the research, Dr Kenneth Setchell, from the Children's Hospital and Medical Centre, Cincinnati, Professor Mark Wahlquist and colleagues, from the Prince Henry Hospital, Melbourne, Dr Knight, from the Royal Hospital for Women, New South Wales, Dr Barnes from the University of Alabama, and Aedin Cassidy, formerly of the University of Surrey. Also an acknowledgement must go to all of the researchers who are quoted in the Reference section.

Next I must thank our patients who were kind enough to share their 'stories' in the text, in the hope that they would be able to help others who were suffering similarly. Despite the fact that they were willing to use their own names, I decided to rename them for the sake of privacy.

As always I am grateful for the support of my team at the WNAS, without whom I would never manage to get the peace of mind to write. I am particularly grateful to our nutritionist, Helen Heap, for her contribution to the menu and recipe section, and for diligently surfing the Internet when I needed extra research data. Thanks also to Gillian Byrne, our nurse, for helping to document the case histories, and to Julie-Anne McWhinnie, a nutritionist visiting from Australia, for her help with updating the research for this new edition and her assistance in interpreting the research on phytoestrogen-rich food values. Cheryl Griffiths, my assistant, as usual kept me going, and discreetly spotted my mistakes.

Thanks are also due to Lavinia Trevor and Charlotte Howard, my literary agents, for their ongoing support and expertise, and to Fiona MacIntyre at Vermilion, for her vision and support.

Special thanks go to my husband, Dr Alan Stewart, who managed the kids when I was missing, cooked me nutritious meals to keep me going, and even cast his eye over the text to check for accuracy. Thanks also to Jackie Hartt and Liz Copping, our 'Deputy Mums', who kept the household ticking over and the children in check. The children would be most miffed if they didn't get a mention for being supportive and helpful. So lastly I humbly thank Phoebe, who particularly demonstrated her excellent culinary skills, Chesney who entertained the kids and perfected his washing-up skills, and Hester and Simeon, who kept me going with their special brand of humour, and lots of kisses and cuddles.

Maryon Stewart
May 2000

INTRODUCTION

The discovery of the health benefits inherently present in phytochemicals is the dawning of a new age for medicine. If taken seriously, it could mean a welcome reduction of the ever increasing statistics for many serious and often fatal diseases, an end to much of the personal suffering that results from pain and illness, and a dramatic reduction in passive suffering whilst watching those near and dear fade away.

I did not personally discover the existence of this wondrous group of substances known as phytochemicals, it was a collective effort by scientists from all around the world. It was they who found the many plant foods that contain the vital ingredients which prevent major diseases and improve the quality of our health. My part was unearthing the discovery as it was being made by scientists all over the world, which probably accounts for my excitement and optimism.

I began reading about the benefits of phytoestrogens for women suffering with menopausal symptoms in the *British Medical Journal* and the *Lancet* in the early 1990s. When I began introducing these important plant substances into our programme at the Women's Nutritional Advisory Service (WNAS) some six years ago, I had absolutely no idea that they would subsequently lead me, with great enthusiasm, on a health education campaign of major proportions.

Throughout the 17 years I have been co-ordinating the activities at the Women's Nutritional Advisory Service it has been our policy to interpret, in ordinary language, the wealth of scientific facts relating to non-drug medicine that have been reported in medical journals by researchers and scientists around the world. The 12 self-help books my husband and I have previously written between us have concentrated on scientifically based self-help measures that people could easily implement to improve their health. Until now our emphasis has been largely placed on nutritional medicine, and how correcting nutritional deficiencies and improving diet and lifestyle help to overcome specific health problems and assist in preventing the long-term health problems that many of us were thought likely to encounter. The phytochemicals, particularly phytoestrogens, around which I have centred this book advance our case considerably. Although they are not classified as nutrients, a massive amount of published research confirms that phytochemicals have incredible powers over our future health prospects.

Despite the fact that according to repeated WNAS surveys, the majority of doctors in the UK, Australia and New Zealand, by their own admission, have little knowledge about the nutritional approach to health, by the 1950s the 13 vitamins that we know today had been discovered. At that point researchers thought that they had pretty much discovered all there was to know about the health properties of foods. There are tens of thousands of medical papers published which verify the scientific basis for the nutritional approach to health and confirm that it is the very foundation of good health. However, since the Second World War the pharmaceutical industry has persuaded doctors and public alike that the drug approach to medicine is far more efficient than relying on foods as a solution to many of our ailments.

If we look back in time, we will see that many famous physicians used foods and herbs to treat ailments long before vitamins and minerals had ever been discovered. Hippocrates, the father of medicine, around 400 BC wrote extensively on the relationship between diet and health. Amongst his recommendations were the use of white willow to treat aches, pains and the pains of childbirth. The white willow tree also provides salicylic acid, which is the active ingredient of the drug we now know as aspirin. Even before Hippocrates, the Greek physician Dioscorides described some 600 plants that had medicinal benefits. Both Plato and Pythagoras advocated a vegetarian diet for health, and Galen, the Greek physician who lived at around 130 AD, outlined the medicinal properties of many foods which subsequently dominated Western medicine for the following 1,500 years.

Before the advent of microscopes and laboratories, the scientists of the world used old-fashioned trial and error. Garlic, for instance, which scientists in recent years have discovered helps to reduce both blood pressure and cholesterol levels, has been used for centuries by civilisations including the Chinese, Greeks, Egyptians, Hebrews, Indians, Japanese and Romans. So it is a fair assumption that this is not a new subject. What is new and exciting, however, is that many of the foods to which we have access in supermarkets and healthfood shops have been blessed with life-saving health properties and modern scientists have been able to confirm these findings in their laboratories.

After 15 years of beating the nutritional medicine drum I have come to know that despite the wealth of published medical studies on the subject of nutrition and herbal medicine, doctors are still not being adequately educated in order to pass on the message to the public. Most postgraduate education for doctors is provided by the pharmaceutical industry, much of which does not have a vested interest in natural remedies. The thousands of medical papers on phytoestrogens, which are published in medical journals all around the world, will probably remain unread by the majority of doctors for many years to come. The purpose of *The Phyto Factor*, therefore, is the dissemination of this newly discovered vital knowledge, with the intention of helping individuals to improve their well-being both in the short and long term, whilst at the same time actively working to prevent many of the diseases that threaten our existence later in life.

Part One, Phytochemicals – The Guardians of Our Health, outlines the key facts and will hopefully answer all the questions about phyto-estrogens you may have, and also help you to assess your individual needs. In Part Two, Eating for Health, you will discover how to meet your needs on a day-by-day basis. There you will find delicious and nutritious menu plans and recipes, which incorporate all the phyto-chemicals and essential nutrients needed for optimum health.

Whilst some enlightened doctors will already be aware of the impor-tance of phytochemicals and will be actively educating their patients, sadly the majority will not for some time to come. The recommenda-tions made in *The Phyto Factor* are all scientifically based, so there is absolutely no need for you to wait to receive the message from your doctor. Study the information and absorb the implications, then use it to improve your own health and that of other family members and friends.

Although the new discoveries contained in *The Phyto Factor* will help you to improve your health, I should point out that these new food secrets should be used in conjunction with other positive dietary and lifestyle changes. Good nutrition and regular exercise are the key to the door to good health; the phytochemicals will improve the quality of what lies behind the door.

It gives me pleasure to enlighten you about the phytochemical family and the valuable role that it plays in human health. Not only do phytochemicals help women over symptoms at the time of the menopause, but also science now confirms they will help to normalise the menstrual cycle, reduce the incidence of hormonally related cancers for men and women, lessen the risk of cardiovascular and heart disease, protect our bones from the bone-thinning disease osteoporosis, lower the incidence of diabetes and keep our skin, hair and nails in tip-top condition. Let us examine why it is that individuals in the Western world badly need to switch on to phytochemicals.

PART ONE

PHYTOCHEMICALS – THE GUARDIANS OF OUR HEALTH

1

WHY WE NEED PHYTOCHEMICALS

Most humans would like to be in the position of knowing that they are actively helping themselves and their families to drastically reduce their risk of many of the killer diseases, including:

- Heart disease
- Cancer of all descriptions
- The bone-thinning disease, osteoporosis
- Diabetes

However, despite the fact that in the Western world we are spending more than ever on food and self-help medication, more of us are getting sick and becoming victims of potentially fatal diseases. In the UK alone we spend £360 million on nutritional and herbal supplements. The alternative health market in the United States is thought to be raking in between $6 billion and $8 billion per year, and in Australia it is in the region of $600 million. In Germany alone, the over-the-counter botanical sales have reached a dizzy $7 billion! Science clearly demonstrates that many of these substances should improve our health, so why is it that statistics for fatal illnesses in Western countries are on the increase, yet remain low in Asian countries? Researchers around the world have set out to answer this question and have discovered that there are underlying secrets, which have thus far eluded us, that hold the key to our health.

During the last decade, the scientific communities have come to realise that discoveries about the health benefits from our diet were not as complete as initially anticipated, but rather still evolving in an exciting way. It was discovered that Mother Nature, in her wisdom, has provided us with foods containing substances that would improve the quality of our health and protect us against many sinister diseases. These potent substances are known as phytochemicals, derived from the Greek word 'phyto', which means plant. It now emerges that they have multiple health benefits including the prevention of osteoporosis, diabetes and kidney disease as well as allowing us to top up our oestrogen levels at the time of the menopause and beyond. There is strong medical evidence to suggest that the daily consumption of certain phytochemicals may also significantly reduce the risk of cancers including breast, cervical, colon, lung, prostate, stomach, uterine cancer and leukaemia. Further benefits of preventing heart and cardiovascular disease and significantly reducing cholesterol levels can be achieved by consuming phytochemicals daily, while at the same time reducing animal protein intake and avoiding certain environmental chemicals.

THE ROLES OF OESTROGEN

Although the hormone oestrogen was first identified in the late 1920s, it is only in recent years that many of its important functions have come to be appreciated amongst medical communities. These include:

- An important role in the formation of the reproductive organs of males and females
- Regulation of menstrual cycles and pregnancies
- Reduction in the risk of heart disease and the bone-thinning disease osteoporosis
- Keeping skin, hair and nails in good shape

If we all had the optimum amount of oestrogen and a healthy diet, consuming nothing that impeded its metabolism, and there was no such thing as the menopause or environmental pollution, we would undoubtedly have better health prospects. The fact is that oestrogen levels fluctuate and are heavily influenced by diet and environmental factors. Too little oestrogen can clearly contribute to major health problems, but so too can an excess. It seems that Western diet and environmental factors hold the key to optimum oestrogen balance. Consider the following astonishing facts:

- In the Japanese language there are no words for the term 'hot flush', largely because women in Japan hardly experience any adverse symptoms at the time of the menopause
- When compared with Western men, whilst a similar number of Japanese men become victims of prostate cancer, far fewer of them actually die as a result. Instead they die as a result of other illnesses or old age, *with* prostate cancer rather than from the cancer itself
- The number of victims of breast cancer and other hormonally related cancer amongst Asians, who consume an Asian diet, is dramatically lower than Western casualties. For example, ten times more

women currently die of breast cancer in England and Wales than in Korea

- Whilst almost half of all Americans die of cardiovascular disease, in Shanghai only one in 15 becomes a victim of cardiovascular disease
- Japanese women have half the hip fracture rate of women in the West, and women in countries like Hong Kong and Singapore suffer even fewer fractures
- Although 50 per cent of some Western populations become victims of diabetes, in other countries diabetes is hardly a health issue.

These somewhat surprising statistics raise a mountain of questions, which scientists around the world are now attempting to answer. It seems that the common denominators of all these facts and figures, are *diet, lifestyle* and *environmental factors*. The Western diet, lifestyle and environment differ so greatly from that of our Asian counterparts that they have reached a point where they are slowly killing us. Although this revelation is understandably depressing, there is good news on the horizon, for it seems that recent research from all over the world has produced enough pieces of the jig-saw puzzle for us to realise that we now have the keys to reverse this trend. The problem is that the wealth of published medical papers that hold the answers are technical, complicated and have not been interpreted into 'normal-speak' for the lay public. As a result, very few people realise that they can seriously influence their health prospects, by relatively simple means.

The message that emerges from the research is exciting and powerful, yet, surprisingly, relatively simple to follow on a day-by-day basis. Essentially there are three key areas we need to address, which are fully explained in Part Two, Eating for Health – The Phyto Factor Diet:

- Consume foods that contain phytochemicals, particularly phyto-estrogens and other cancer-preventing foods like anti-oxidants, daily. Oranges, for example, contain 170 different phytochemicals that protect our health, and soya products are amongst the richest sources of naturally occurring oestrogen
- Reduce intake of animal fat to a minimum, and replace it with good oils that contain essential fatty acids that protect us against heart disease and cancer
- Take steps to avoid contacting and consuming environmental chemicals where possible.

It really is not an onerous regime and there is an enormous amount of scientific evidence to support each of its aspects. Changing habits of a lifetime may not necessarily be an easy task to undertake, but the pay-off in health terms is so great that it will be a sound investment of effort. Phytoestrogen-rich food alone has been shown by exceedingly reputable scientists to have some remarkable effects on the cells of the body and on many of its organs. Just a few of the amazing feats phytochemicals have been able to perform include:

- Turning cancer cells back into normal healthy cells
- Unblocking clogged arteries
- Helping to generate new bone, thus protecting bone mass
- Normalising blood sugar, thus helping to control diabetes
- Dramatically reducing hot flushes at the time of the menopause
- Regulating the menstrual cycle

These new research findings mean that we now have a choice about preserving our health. If you have come this far, I presume you are keen to learn about phytochemicals, what they are, how they perform these miracles, and which foods are rich sources.

2

THE FAMILY OF PHYTOCHEMICALS – MOTHER NATURE'S SECRETS

Many common plant-based foods and herbs contain powerful substances known as phytochemicals. There are hundreds of active compounds, which largely fall into the following categories:

PHYTOCHEMICALS:

Phytoestrogens – the main classes of phytoestrogen are
• Isoflavones
• Lignans
• Coumestans
• Resorclic acid lactones

There are several types of isoflavones: genistein, daidzein, glycetein, formononetin and biochanin A. The main lignans are matairesinol and secoisolariciresinol, while the main coumestan is coumestrol.

The University of Minnesota highlighted some additional classes of phytochemicals that also show anti-cancer activity:

Allium compounds – found mainly in onions, garlic and chives
Coumarins – found in vegetables and citrus fruit
Dithiolthiones – present in cruciferous vegetables including broccoli, Brussels sprouts, cabbage and cauliflower
Flavonoids – in most fruits and vegetables
Glucosinolates, indoles – also found in cruciferous vegetables
Glyceritinic acid – found in liquorice (but this can have adverse effects on blood pressure) (see page 93)
Inositol hexaphosphate – present in plants, particularly soya beans and cereals
Isothiocyanates, thiocyanates – in cruciferous vegetables
Limonene – from citrus fruits.

Current science tells us a little about each of these groups, but as the years roll by, we will undoubtedly be learning more about their health benefits.

WHAT ARE PHYTOESTROGENS?

These wondrous substances can be found in common foods including the soya bean, chickpeas, lentils and a whole host of vegetables, nuts, seeds and berries. The four main isoflavones are genistein, daidzein, formononetin and biochanin. They are not nutrients, but they have a marked effect on our health.

Although phytoestrogens are similar in structure to the female hormone oestrogen, they are only 1/1000th as potent. Despite this, research now shows that they protect us against hormonally related cancers as they have the ability to block the uptake of excess oestrogen by the body, and even raise low levels when necessary. It seems that they mimic oestrogen's role in the body and are able to compete successfully for the receptor sites at the entrance to cells. So, for example, genistein, the look-alike oestrogen, is able successfully to take up occupation in breast tissue, thus preventing the more potent natural oestrogen from converting normal cells into cancerous cells. (See the relationship between HRT and breast cancer on page 80). High oestrogen levels are also associated with female cancers of the breast, cervix, ovaries and uterus, and prostate cancer in men. Some 300 plants are thought to contain phytoestrogens, with soya beans, linseeds (flaxseeds), chickpeas and lentils being the richest sources.

Genistein

This is a compound found only in soya, and is the most extensively studied isoflavone to-date. Although it was identified as a plant oestrogen in 1966, it took over 20 years for its anti-cancer properties to be recognised by the medical profession. Japanese researchers first discovered that genistein was capable of blocking the signal that triggers the growth of a cancer cell, and that it was also able to inhibit the growth of cancerous tumours.

Because genistein is able to block the uptake of oestrogen it acts as an 'anti-oestrogen', in a similar way to the drug tamoxifen administered to breast cancer victims, but without any side-effects. It prevents the growth of cancer cells by inhibiting the activity of oncogenes, the genes that promote cancer, and other cancer-causing enzymes, which activate the development of certain types of cancer. It even seems to

18

have the ability to reverse the intention of a cancer cell causing cancer cells to change back to normal cells. Also it is able to block the blood supply to a cancerous tumour, which results in the tumour dying due to starvation. Whilst performing all these miracles it also acts as a powerful anti-oxidant, protecting cells from free radical attack which comes from radiation and chemical pollutants, without inhibiting the growth of normal cells.

By the early 1990s Professor Herman Adlercreutz, one of the key researchers in this area, had clearly established that Japanese men, who consume soya products on a regular basis, had plasma levels of isoflavones more than 100 times higher than their Finnish counterparts. At around this time it was also discovered that Japanese men, whilst having a similar rate of prostate cancer to Western fellows, instead of dying as a result of it, die with it. In other words the cancer grows so slowly that it does not impinge on their longevity. (See section on prostate cancer on page 106.)

We have reached the point where some researchers believe that genistein should be included in the treatment of most cancers. In one study conducted at the University of Minnesota, genistein successfully managed to destroy leukaemia cells in mice.

Other studies have shown that genistein has a role in reducing the oestrogen withdrawal symptoms associated with the menopause, including hot flushes, night sweats, dry vagina and insomnia, and in the prevention of osteoporosis. It also has the ability to inhibit platelet aggregation, which means it prevents blood cells from clumping together, thus reducing the incidence of heart attacks, strokes and the development of atherosclerosis (furring of the arteries). As well as all this, it has anti-inflammatory properties, which means that it may also be helpful in reducing arthritis and other rheumatic diseases.

Daidzein

This is the other main isoflavone found in soya, which has been found to be beneficial to us in a similar way to genistein. Like genistein it acts as both an anti-cancer agent and an anti-oxidant. It also has a role to play in the prevention of bone mass depletion and once again is able to cause cancer cells to revert to normal.

Formononetin and Biochanin A

These are two of the four major oestrogenic isoflavones which are chiefly derived from red clover, chickpeas, lentils and mung beans. Formononetin, a methylated daidzein, and biochanin, a methylated genistein, have unique effects on human physiology that are not possessed by the non-methylated isoflavones genistein and daidzein found in soya. The data suggests that they appear to be superior agents which may be more effective as cancer-protective compounds. They are also reported to be responsible for the positive lipid (blood fat) lowering properties associated with traditional diets.

Isoflavones in general seem to have a normalising effect on our hormones. We have looked at how they block the absorption of an excess of oestrogen, but, amazingly, they are also able to raise oestrogen levels in women whose levels are low. There is evidence to show that they help to regulate the menstrual cycle (see page 76), which makes them desirable to women of all ages.

Glyroside and Glycitein

These are the most recently discovered isoflavones and also demonstrate some of the benefits of genistein and daidzein. Other types include formononetin, biochanin A and coumestrol.

Lignans

Like soya products, lignans possess both weak oestrogenic and antioestrogenic qualities, and are structurally similar to oestradiol (a form of oestrogen). In humans, lignans including Secoisolariciresinol (Seco) and Matairesinol (Mat), which are derived mainly from linseeds (flaxseeds), are converted from Matairesinol and secoisolariciresinol, by intestinal bacteria to hormone-like compounds enterolactone and enterodiol respectively. When linseeds are consumed, intestinal bacterial action results in the production of up to 800 times more of these lignans than from any other food. They have a positive effect on sex hormone production, metabolism, growth, biological and enzyme function, and to some degree, have a protective effect against some forms of cancer, particularly breast cancer. More research is needed to determine just how lignans modulate oestrogen metabolism and their role in breast cancer prevention.

Coumestans

The main type of coumestan is coumestrol. The richest food sources are mung-bean sprouts and alfalfa sprouts. Coumestrol has been shown to compete with oestrogen for receptor sites in breast tumour cells. It has also been shown to have anti-oxidant properties, and the ability to prevent further growth of cancer cells.

Phenolic acids

These compounds have anti-oxidant properties and prevent cells from being attacked by carcinogens (cancer-causing substances). Rich sources are grapes, red wine, tea, citrus and other fruits and vegetables.

Phytates – phytic acid

Until fairly recently, phytic acid was considered to be a substance to be avoided because of its ability to impede the absorption of important minerals like iron, calcium and zinc. However, more recent research has caused the medical profession to regard phytic acid in a new light because of its valuable anti-oxidant properties. The anti-oxidant properties appear to enhance our immunity as they are able to bind with iron in the intestines. In the presence of oxygen, iron can create 'free radicals', which are able to attack our DNA. By binding with iron, phytic acid is able to prevent the creation of free radicals by keeping the iron away from the oxygen. The result is the control of free radicals which results in the reduction of risk of heart disease possibly caused by high iron levels in post-menopausal women, some men and those with the rare blood condition, haemocromotosis. Phytic acid has also been shown to help prevent some cancers, including breast and colon cancer, as well as reducing the incidence of heart and cardiovascular disease. Good sources are plants, particularly soya products and cereals.

Phytosterols

These have been shown to inhibit the development of cancers including colon and skin cancer, and may also help to prevent heart disease by helping to control cholesterol levels. Like the omega-3 essential fatty acids they contain anti-inflammatory properties, and additionally are needed for muscle stamina and strength. Good sources are vegetables, including soya beans.

Protease inhibitors

This is another compound that has been re-examined by the medical profession. At one time protease inhibitors were thought to promote cancer, whereas now it seems that they have the ability to inhibit the action of enzymes that stimulate the growth of a cancerous tumour. Soya contains a unique protease inhibitor known as the Bowman-Birk Inhibitor (BBI), which appears to be a key compound in the inhibition of tumour growth. Dr Ann Kennedy, of the University of Pennsylvania School of Medicine, conducted a study which involved adding BBI to the diet of rats who had previously been fed a substance that was known to cause colon cancer. She was able to bring about a 100 per cent reduction in the formation of tumours. Another similar study on mice suppressed the formation of tumours by 71 per cent. As well as helping to inhibit a wide range of cancers, including cancer of the colon, lung, oesophagus, pancreas and mouth, they have also been found to prevent the activation of specific genes that cause cancer. Additionally, they protect cells from the damaging effects of environmental pollution and radiation. Good sources are most plants, particularly seeds and legumes such as soya beans.

Saponins

Like phytates, saponins have anti-oxidant properties that protect us from the damaging effects of free radicals as well as helping to control cholesterol. One study showed that they directly inhibited colon cancer and another showed that when mixed with HIV virus they stopped the virus from growing. Good sources are plants, particularly soya beans.

THE DOOR TO HEALTH

There is a wealth of evidence to support the fact that the groups of foods outlined in this section have a major influence on the health prospects of people all over the world. We have been spoiled for choice in the latter part of the twentieth century, and our increased prosperity has encouraged us to veer off the nutritional tracks and make poor choices. Consequently, our consumption of animal fat, sugar, salt and prepared processed foods has increased dramatically, whilst our intake of more wholesome options like pulses, nuts, seeds and vegetables has fallen. Obesity has doubled in recent years, bringing with it many unforeseen health problems. The discovery of these powerful phyto-chemicals gives us the key to the door to health. If we backtrack, taking care to follow a nutritional diet rich in many of the phyto-chemicals, we will undoubtedly be able not only to improve our own health prospects, but also that of our families. Now let us compare the different types of oestrogen and the effect that each has on the body.

3

SYNTHETIC OESTROGEN VS. PHYTOESTROGEN

Unlike the naturally occurring oestrogen found in food, the environmental oestrogens, known as xenoestrogens, 'xeno' being the Greek word for foreign, are far from beneficial to health. Horror story reports about xenoestrogens have been widespread in the media in the last few years, telling tales of reduced sperm counts in men and infertility, and even increased rates of oestrogen-related cancers.

ENVIRONMENTAL OESTROGENS DEFINED

Some 37 chemicals have been identified as being able to mimic oestrogen in the body and, although they are weaker than natural oestrogen, they are thought to interfere with the systems that regulate the production of oestrogen and sex hormone function generally. Many of these 'xenoestrogens', or 'ecoestrogens' as they are sometimes known, are produced by industry for specific purposes including use in pesticides, plastics and electrical transformers. These include chlorinated hydrocarbon, the insecticide DDT and its breakdown product DDE, and a number of polychlorinated biphenyls (PCBs), dioxins and several fungicides, and some of the chemicals used in detergents and plastics. Other xenoestrogens are produced as a by-product of manufacturing processes, or result from the breakdown products of other chemicals.

A study of Florida alligators inhabiting DDE-polluted rivers revealed low rates of hatching, and those eggs that did hatch were predominantly female offspring, or males with abnormally small penises. Male Texan turtles whose shells, prior to hatching, had been exposed to oestrogen-mimicking chemicals, developed ovaries.

Besides these examples, there have been a number of other animal studies that have revealed reproductive abnormalities following exposure to environmental chemicals. Many scientists now also believe that repeated exposure to these xenoestrogens is related to the increased risk of breast tumours in women.

THE DIFFERENCES EXPLAINED

The problem with many of these environmental substances is that they do not biodegrade in the same way as naturally occurring oestrogens, instead they collect in the fatty tissues of the body. Natural oestrogens are broken down in the body within anything from minutes to hours, after which they are broken into pieces by liver enzymes and either flushed out as waste, or reused to build other molecules.

Most of the phytoestrogens that we consume in our diets are absorbed into the body. The process of absorption requires that they undergo a variety of changes. Our stomach acid, bacteria in our bowels and the liver, which is the 'clearing house' of the body, all make structural changes to the phytoestrogens. Once metabolised by the body only a small amount of these compounds can be identified as the original plant compound, the majority will be converted from plant to human compounds. These new compounds, being water soluble, are free to circulate throughout the body having access to every cell, and like other hormones in the body are gradually filtered out through the urine.

In the same way, phytoestrogens are easily broken down by our bodies and are not stored in the fatty tissue. Following consumption they are either flushed out of the body intact, or are broken down and changed in the body so that they can act like oestrogens. Conversely, the synthetic xenoestrogens hang around. They are not easily broken down and whilst some are flushed out by the body, many remain intact either in the environment or, as most of them are lipophilic, which means that they prefer to be surrounded by fat cells rather than water, they collect in the fatty tissue of both human and animal bodies where they remain for years.

As well as collecting in our fat stores, xenoestrogens are present in the water supply and much of our plant food is exposed to them as a result of farming or environmental factors. They collect in the food chain like panthers waiting to pounce. We know that they are able to cross the placenta to developing babies, and although there is no conclusive evidence to show that they affect human development, wildlife and laboratory animal studies are pointing to the fact that many of these chemicals may indeed be detrimental to development in the reproductive phase. Research so far points to the fact that during pregnancy, breastfeeding or episodes of stress, these xenoestrogens can be released from the fat cells and either passed on to offspring, or redistributed.

How xenoestrogens differ

The chemical structure of environmental oestrogens is strikingly different from both oestrogen found in the body and oestrogen found in plants. Natural oestrogen consists of chains of carbon rings differing only in location and number of attachments to the main stem, whereas environmental oestrogens come in literally all shapes and sizes. These structural differences may well account for the functional differences. The normal habit of the oestrogen that we manufacture in our bodies is to use the bloodstream as its mode of transport while it hunts out compatible receptor sites, which are located in the nucleus of cells. Oestrogen then enters the cell and forms a relationship with the receptor like a hand in a glove. This stimulates our genes to send chemical messages to other parts of our cells with instructions to change the way in which the cell functions, for example to produce more of an enzyme, to divide or to grow. So at around the time of ovulation each month, when a new egg is released from the ovary, oestrogen will bind with receptor sites inside the cells of the uterus with the specific purpose of encouraging the lining of the uterus to grow thicker in preparation for a developing embryo.

Synthetic environmental oestrogens can also interact directly with the receptor sites within the cells, but the outcome is usually different, in that they can block normal hormone activity. Current theories regarding the possible actions of xenoestrogens are that they can perform a number of functions varying from mimicking a proper hormone response, to inhibiting the normal response completely, or even a bit of both. They can even bind to other receptors and cause a completely different response, all of which may well change our hormonal blood concentrations and responses as a result.

POTENTIAL LONG-TERM EFFECTS

Shortly after the beginning of the Second World War, we began using chemicals on a wide scale. Developing babies who have been exposed to many of these chemicals during their developmental phase would not have reached maturity until the 1970s. The extent to which children born towards the end of the twentieth century have been affected may not become apparent for many years because some of the consequences of exposure may not be evident for some 20 to 40 years after birth.

Synthetic oestrogen, ethinyl oestradiol, used in many preparations of the oral contraceptive pill, also appears in small concentrations in water supplies. This has been another area of concern in recent years, but the synthetic oestrogens are not as persistent as the xenoestrogens. Another form of synthetic oestrogen, diethylstilbestrol (DES), was widely used as a growth promoter in animals from the 1950s until the 1980s when it was banned, although it is still used in some places to control malaria. From 1948 to 1971 DES was also prescribed in both the USA and the UK to over five million women who were diagnosed as having low oestrogen levels. It was later confirmed that daughters of these women had a high risk of developing rare vaginal cancers and their sons had an increased risk of sexual abnormalities including malformed penises, abnormally small testes, low sperm counts and, in the worst cases, testicular cancer.

A review of 61 medical papers on semen quality was published by a Danish professor in the *British Medical Journal* in 1992, concluding that there had been a dramatic 50 per cent decline in sperm counts in men world-wide since 1940. More recent European studies indicate that the quality of sperm is declining as well as the quantity, and that men born after 1950 are more likely to be affected. The incidence of testicular cancer has also doubled in Western countries over the last 50 years, to the point where it is the most common cancer experienced by young men. During this same period it has been observed that defects of the male reproductive tract have also increased.

Organochlorine pesticides

An incredible scenario occurred in Israel, which made me gasp for breath. Israel has had astronomical levels of breast cancer cases to deal with for many years. However, in 1990, two environmental specialists from the Hebrew University's Hadassah School of Medicine discovered to their amazement that the number of deaths from breast cancer fell sharply between 1976 and 1986. This was in spite of per capita risks being on the increase, like increased intake of animal fats and delayed pregnancy. Instead of the 20 per cent rise in statistics that they expected, there was a 34 per cent drop, amounting to a difference of over 50 per cent. Westin and Richter, the two scientists, eventually connected the dramatic fall in death from breast cancer to a 1978 Israeli ban on the use of three organochlorine pesticides, alpha-benzene hexachloride (BHC), gamma benzene hexachloride (lindane) and DDT, which had previously been used extensively in Israeli cowsheds. Milk and other dairy products in Israel had previously been contaminated with these pesticides at rates of between 100 and 1,000 times greater than levels found in the USA, which resulted in public outcry and the subsequent ban in Israel.

Animal experiments conducted in the 1960s had shown that organochlorine pesticides caused breast cancer in rats, and in 1981 one research study concluded that these pesticides might be considered possible contributors to the high incidence of breast cancer amongst women. Critics were quick to challenge the Israeli findings, claiming that environmentally induced cancers take at least 20 years to develop. However, as organochlorine pesticides are 'complete' carcinogens, which are able to initiate and promote tumour growth, they are able to change cancer statistics quite rapidly. Recent German research has clearly demonstrated a link between organochlorines and breast cancer. They discovered a two-fold increase in breast cancer among female workers who had been exposed to dioxin contamination at a chemical plant in Hamburg. Other American studies on chemical workers, including professional chemists and hairdressers, have also shown a dramatic increase in the death rate from breast cancer.

Analyses of breast tissue have since taken place, and indeed, in one study, the biopsied breast tissue of a woman with breast cancer contained 40 per cent more chlorinated pesticides than tissue from women whose biopsies proved negative. Another study, published in the *Journal of the National Cancer Institute* in 1993, discovered that the blood from women who later developed breast cancer registered much higher levels of DDE, effectively meaning that they had up to four times greater risk of developing breast cancer.

One would assume that following these alarming findings an international ban on organochlorine pesticides would have been quickly initiated. Nevertheless, to date this has not been forthcoming. Consequently, we are left to wonder whether the reluctance to ban these pesticides may have any bearing on the fact that much of the ongoing cancer research is funded by the very same companies who are manufacturing the organochlorine pesticides!

As well as being toxic, organochlorides mimic oestrogen and, when in competition with ordinary oestrogen, have the ability to compete for the receptor sites within the cells. Once connected they trigger various undesirable changes in the body. This must be the most worrying scenario relating to our chances of becoming cancer victims, and not one we should accept. Addresses of the campaigning organisations like Greenpeace and Breast Cancer Action can be found in the Useful Addresses Section starting on page 259, and I'm sure they would like some extra support. In the meantime, there are a number of ways we can avoid xenoestrogens, and these are listed in the checklist at the end of the chapter.

CONCLUSION

There is a large body of data supporting the hypothesis that environmental oestrogens may be detrimental to human health. Equally, there is data to support the opposite argument. However, absence of evidence is not evidence of absence, and further research should be a priority. It is interesting to note that in the last 60 years since the first report that a number of man-made chemicals were oestrogenic, there have been changes in the age of onset of puberty, and increases in hormone-modulated diseases and disorders such as breast and prostate cancer, and polycystic ovarian disease.

PHYTOESTROGENS – SOME BETTER NEWS

What comes over loudly and clearly from numerous research papers is that phytoestrogens, the oestrogens that occur naturally in our food and in plants, are able to compete *successfully* for the receptor sites within the body. With Mother Nature guiding them, not only are they able to raise oestrogen levels in those whose levels are in need of a boost, but they are also able to block the absorption of high levels of oestrogen within the body, both natural and environmental. As you will see from later chapters, it seems that they have enormous healing powers and are even able to persuade a cancer cell to return to being a normal healthy cell.

SELF-HELP MEASURES TO AVOID XENOESTROGENS

The constant bombardment by environmental oestrogen is obviously an area of great concern for us all, and an issue that is currently out of our control to a large degree. There are, however, a number of steps that we can take to protect ourselves from many of the chemical pitfalls, thus increasing our health prospects; the diet detailed in Part Two has been designed to help you achieve this. In the meantime, there are a few self-help tips for your consideration:

- Whenever possible, buy organic food. It is often available from health food shops, some supermarkets and local farms. Box schemes are a convenient way of having organic produce delivered to your door. See page 250 for a Product Directory. Or, if you have the opportunity, grow your own fruit and vegetables

- If you eat meat, buy additive free meat, and trim the excess fat away before cooking, as the xenoestrogens accumulate in the fat
- Restrict your intake of animal fat to a complete minimum, and use wholesome oils containing essential fatty acids
- Store food in plastic-free containers
- Use plastic-free cling-film to cover your left-overs
- Lose weight if you are overweight, as in common with animals we store xenoestrogens in our fatty tissue
- Use filtered tap water or bottled water
- Purchase non-bleached paper products, including coffee filters, toilet tissue, kitchen roll and stationery
- Refrain from using pesticides or herbicides in your garden
- Consume as much in the way of foods containing phytoestrogens as you possibly can, as these types of oestrogen seem to compete successfully for the receptor sites in the body, reducing the negative effects of other forms of oestrogen
- Use tampons and sanitary towels that are produced without chlorine
- Use alternatives to chlorine-based bleach for household chores
- Avoid aerosols, including anti-perspirants and hair spray
- If possible, use alternatives to the oral contraceptive pill or Hormone Replacement Therapy.

4

PROTEIN: ANIMAL VS. PLANT

Until now the soya bean has been exceedingly underrated in prosperous circles and even considered to be a second-class protein. In fact many omnivores have been brought up to regard animal products as the standard dietary protein, and it is therefore only educated vegetarians and a minority of adventurous individuals in the Western world who have included the soya bean in their diet in a serious way thus far. Ironically, in poorer countries around the world where plant-based foods predominate in the diet due to lack of funds, conditions like heart disease and cancer are far less of a problem. And in Japan and other Asian countries where the soya bean is the favoured protein in the diet, the incidence of these fatal diseases is dramatically lower.

Amino acids

We all need to consume protein on a daily basis, as it is needed for tissue growth and repair. Protein is a string or strings of amino acids, which are our building blocks. Our diet is composed of some 20 amino acids which, when digested, break down into individual amino acids and are subsequently converted to provide the body with the enzymes and antibodies that it requires. We are able to manufacture 11 of the 20 amino acids within the body without having to rely on our diet. The remaining nine, known as essential amino acids, must be obtained from our diet. One of the functions of amino acids is to supply nitrogen, which is essential to the body, but is not found in other nutrients. If we fail to consume sufficient protein to replace the amount of nitrogen we lose through our waste products daily, the body will be unable to function.

HOW VEGETABLE AND ANIMAL PROTEIN COMPARE

Animal protein usually provides the full range of amino acids needed by the body, and for this reason it has come to be regarded as an easy and sensible option. Plant proteins, as a general rule, tend to be short of some of the essential amino acids, and unless eaten in combination with other vegetable proteins, or at least consumed on the same day, will not supply the complete range of amino acids. The most commonly missing amino acid is known as the 'limiting amino acid'. Proteins have to be broken down into amino acids by enzymes before they can be used by the body, and once again animal proteins look more attractive as they are slightly more digestible than vegetarian protein.

The average adult should aim to consume 0.8 gram of protein each day per kilogram (2.2 lb) of body weight, which is a figure that has been set on the high side to compensate for those whose protein needs are high. Therefore, you can calculate your needs by dividing the number of pounds you weigh by 2.2 to determine your kilogram weight, and then multiply the figure by 0.8 to get your answer. If you weigh 63 kilos (140 lb) your daily protein requirement will be in the region of 50 grams. Although people are often concerned about getting sufficient protein, the truth is that most of us consume considerably more than we require each day, with some Americans consuming almost double their requirements. Protein requirements vary for certain groups of people including children, body builders and pregnant women by between 10 and 20 per cent.

Many civilisations have existed in good health on combinations of plant food for centuries. Their secret has been the combination of foods in order to get their complete amino acid requirements. In the Middle East, chickpeas and sesame seeds are often eaten together to make a complete protein, in Asia the tendency is to combine soya beans and rice to achieve the same goal, African communities often combine corn with nuts and beans, and in Thailand peanuts and rice are often found together on the menu.

Although it is possible to get an adequate protein intake from vegetarian sources alone, it is not essential, unless you are contemplating switching to a complete vegetarian diet or, of course, if you already follow a vegetarian diet. The diet detailed in Part Two of *The Phyto Factor* is designed to encourage you to include as many of the phytoestrogens in your diet as possible, but it is not exclusively vegetarian. I have included vegetarian options, so it will be up to you to choose those that you find most palatable.

THE AMAZING SOYA BEAN

The soya bean, which is known in China as 'ta-tou' meaning the 'greater bean' and is referred to in America as 'the miracle bean', has been shown to be at least an equivalent source of protein to animal products. Its amino acid content matches well with human requirements, and it is well digested. According to the researchers Virginia and Mark Messina, the digestibility of the various soya products is as follows:

- Soya protein – including textured vegetarian protein (TVP) – 95 per cent digestible
- Tofu – 92 per cent digestible
- Soya flour – 85–90 per cent digestible
- Only toasted or steamed whole soya beans are poorly digested.

Soya products are also a good source of fibre and important nutrients including B vitamins, the minerals calcium, iron and zinc. The soya bean has a higher fat content than most other plant foods, but still has a considerably lower saturated fat content than animal products, and unlike animal products contains no cholesterol. Although soya oil and the fat in soya foods contain approximately 15 per cent saturated fat they also contain polyunsaturated and mono-unsaturated fats. Soya is one of the few plants that contains omega-3 essential fatty acids, which are usually found in marine fish oils and are thought to be helpful in the prevention of heart disease and cancer. Research shows that these omega-3s are also needed for brain development in growing infants.

Soya beans were first discovered by Chinese farmers in Asia over 5,000 years ago, and according to Chinese tradition are one of the five sacred crops that were named by the emperor of the time, Sheng-Nung. Tofu, which is made from curdled soya milk, is thought to have been developed by Buddhist monks in approximately 164 BC. The popularity of soya products slowly spread across Asia, but it wasn't until approximately the 1800s that they arrived in Europe. Soya products have become so popular in China that the milkman even makes his round delivering soya milk; at one point soya milk sales outsold Coca-Cola! Liquid squeezed from soya beans has been used traditionally to make tea by the elderly, to treat kidney diseases, the common cold, skin diseases, diarrhoea, anaemia, constipation, toxaemia in pregnancy and to stimulate milk production in breastfeeding mothers.

By 1920, Dr John Harvey Kellogg, the founder of the Kellogg's company who was a keen vegetarian, began marketing the first soya-based breakfast cereal and soya milk. Another doctor excited about the health properties of soya was Dr Horvath, who became known as the 'Father of Soya' in the USA, and later established what is now known as the American Soya Bean Association.

Today over 50 million metric tons of soya beans, which is approximately half the world's crop, are produced each year in America. While approximately one third is shipped to Japan where it becomes an integral part of the diet, 90–95 per cent of the remaining crop is used as animal feed rather than for human consumption. This trend will undoubtedly change once the word is out that it has been demonstrated beyond all doubt that soya products have incredible health properties. You will see this in the next few chapters, which deal with individual conditions.

The power of linseeds

The organically grown golden linseed is a greatly underestimated product that in fact has a great deal going for it. It comes in the form of little seeds about double the size of sesame seeds. It is sometimes referred to as 'flaxseed' and is more widely known for its oil, which is used to protect cricket bats and is a constituent of paint and varnish. As well as the linseeds themselves, which have a wealth of health benefits, the cold-pressed organic linseed oil, which is prepared for human consumption, is probably the richest source of omega-3 oils and is sometimes referred to as 'nutritional gold'. Linseeds contain 100–800 times more plant lignans than their closest competitors, wheat, rye, soya, oats, millet or buckwheat. Lignans are thought to be oestrogen modulators which have the ability to lower or raise oestrogen levels. The Latin name for linseed is *Linum usitatissimum*, which means 'extremely useful', and indeed it is. Although linseeds have existed for over 5,000 years, it is only in recent years that their health properties have been recognised. Cherokee Indians regarded linseed as being as sacred as the eagle feather, believing that it captured energies from the sun that were vital to the life process. They used it to increase male virility, to nourish pregnant women and even for healing arthritis and skin diseases. In modern times cold-pressed linseed oil is used by athletes to increase their stamina and recovery time. Flour derived from linseed is also being used increasingly in bread and bakery products to provide not only a nutty flavour, but also to increase the nutritional and health benefits of the final product.

Why are essential fatty acids so important?

Linseeds are rich sources of two very important compounds, linoleic acid (LA) and alpha-linolenic acid (ALA), which are included in the list of nutrients that the body cannot produce. Omega-3 fatty acids can be found in seeds and plants from cold climates, green leafy vegetables and in cold-water oily fish including mackerel, herring, salmon, sardines, pilchards, tuna and cod. The modern diet is lacking in essential fatty acids, and more than 60 illnesses and health problems have been linked to fatty acid abnormalities. In fact, researchers now believe that deficiency of omega-3 has caused as much illness as scurvy did before the discovery of vitamin C deficiency. Despite this, and the fact that many of the world's civilisations once regarded linseed as having both healing and nourishing properties, many supermarkets do not stock either linseed oil or seeds.

Signs and symptoms of omega-3 deficiency

- Behavioural changes
- Dry skin
- Elevated levels of trigly-cerides (blood fats)
- Growth retardation
- High blood pressure
- Impaired learning ability
- Impaired vision

- Immune dysfunction
- Lack of co-ordination
- Low metabolic rate
- Mental deterioration
- Tingling in arms and legs
- Tissue inflammation
- Sticky platelets (red blood cells)
- Water retention

One of the reasons why supermarkets are reluctant to stock linseeds or linseed oil, and much of our food is stripped of the omega-3 compo-nents, is because of their short shelf life. The alpha linolenic acid, which is a member of the omega-3 essential fatty acid group, becomes rancid quickly once it has made contact with oxygen, to which it is highly attracted. Ironically, the fact that the omega-3s attract oxygen is an advantage to our health as they play a key role in carrying oxygen around the body. Apart from the fact that food processing removes the omega-3s, whatever omega-3 remains is then usually destroyed through the hydrogenation process. If you read most margarine labels for exam-ple, you will come across the term 'hydrogenated', which means that hydrogen has been added to change unsaturated oils into saturated, thus producing a longer shelf life. The hydrogenation process makes liquid hard at room temperature.

As well as alpha linolenic acid, another essential fatty acid is linole-ic acid. This is part of the omega-6 family, and is another nutrient of vital importance to human health, which once again needs to be obtained from our diet as it cannot be manufactured within the body. Rich sources are sunflower, safflower and corn oils, many unsalted nuts, excluding peanuts, and seeds, plus green vegetables. Linoleic acid, omega-6, is also present in linseeds, 16 per cent compared to omega-3's 55 per cent content. This is good news, as our modern diet tends to deliver up to 25 times more omega-6 than omega-3, and for optimum health they should be consumed in balance.

Signs and symptoms of omega-6 deficiency

- Arthritis
- Circulation and heart disorders
- Dry skin
- Eczema
- Hair loss
- Liver and kidney problems
- Lowered immunity
- Sterility

The consequence of raising essential fatty acid levels with the consumption of linseeds or cold-pressed linseed oil, is that the body can then perform the biological functions that require optimum levels of essential fatty acids (EFAs). This has a knock-on effect which results in the resolution or at least improvement of many health problems. Some of the health benefits of essential fatty acids include:

- Helping to regulate cholesterol metabolism
- Helping to control inflammation
- Maintaining and regulating the functions of all cell membranes, which are mostly made of fat
- Serving as precursors to the very active hormone-like substances known as prostaglandins, which regulate nearly every body function
- Reduction of hot flushes at the time of the menopause, and the regeneration of the lining of the vagina as a result of the oestrogenic and anti-inflammatory properties
- Regulation of the menstrual cycle to a normal length
- Reducing blood cholesterol levels (LDLs)
- Reducing blood fat levels associated with heart attacks and strokes
- Reducing incidence of colon and breast cancer
- Improving skin quality
- Reducing the incidence of depression and mental illness
- Reducing symptoms of arthritis
- Prevention of allergies
- Helping to counteract immune disorders
- And, last, but not least, they are a brilliant cure for constipation and are helpful with colon cleansing and healing a leaky gut.

The benefits of red clover

Red clover is another hot contender in the phytoestrogen stakes. It is a member of the leguminosae family, and is a nitrogen-fixing plant with numerous varieties. It has been widely used as a soil-improving crop, to enrich the nitrogen levels in the soil. It is a native crop of Europe and the temperate regions of Central and Northern Asia, northwest Africa and Australia. It is one of the world's oldest agricultural crops, used as a source of hay for cattle, horses and sheep and a source of nectar for bees in summer. It has also been used for centuries as a medicinal herb. The Chinese have long used an infusion of the flowers as an expectorant and the Russians traditionally have used infusions for bronchial asthma. Other cultures have used it to treat anything from sore eyes to digestive distress, psoriasis and eczema. It is particularly rich in isoflavones, and is a unique source of formononetin and biochanin.

Each legume type has a different isoflavone profile. Soya has only daidzein and genistein; some varieties of chickpeas have predominantly formononetin and biochanin whilst others have predominantly genistein and daidzein. In Mediterranean countries, Latin America and India, the methylated isoflavones dominate in Asian countries, the non-methylated isoflavones because of the widespread use of soya, but these communities still receive all four isoflavones in their diet through their use of other legumes such as aduki, lab-lab and mung beans.

Early researchers thought that the methylated isoflavones were fully demethylated by humans. This meant that it didn't matter if your diet contained methylated or non-methylated isoflavones – the end result would still be only daidzein and genistein in the blood. Research by Novogen, the manufacturers of Red Clover, has shown this to be incorrect. Humans do have demethylation capacity, by the liver, but this is incomplete. So all communities have all four oestrogenic isoflavones in their blood. According to the Novogen research each of the four oestrogenic isoflavones has a particular biological profile. For example, biochanin is about ten times more active as an anti-oestrogen than its derivative genistein, a property that might be quite relevant when it comes to the anti-cancer protective effect of the isoflavones on breast tissue. Also, formononetin appears to be the principally active isoflavone on cholesterol metabolism.

If we are to derive the full range of biological benefits from dietary isoflavones, then it would seem important to obtain all four oestrogenic isoflavones in the diet. This means either eating a variety of legumes including soya, chick peas and lentils, to ensure a spread of isoflavones, or using a supplement like Novogen Red Clover, see page 70, which is the only supplement currently on the market capable of delivering blood levels of all four isoflavones at levels and in proportions similar to that of vegetarians.

Whilst animals that have grazed in pastures containing concentrated amounts of clover have subsequently experienced reproductive problems and infertility, studies on humans have not reached the same conclusions. In fact the human studies to date, using moderate levels of red clover, have found only beneficial effects.

CAN WE OVERDOSE ON ISOFLAVONES?

Scientists are wary about overdosing on phytoestrogens, as the long-term effect of high doses has not been studied. Some of the key studies that have been undertaken used doses of between 40 mg and 60 mg of isoflavones daily. Dr John Eden and his colleagues at the Royal Hospital for Women in New South Wales (Australia) used 160 mg of isoflavones daily for three months and recorded a significant reduction in several menopausal symptoms, particularly hot flushes. At Tufts University in Boston researchers used a soya bar containing 40 mg per day of isoflavones and recorded a small decrease in menopausal symptoms over 12 weeks. Dr Harding and colleagues, who conducted a proper double-blind cross-over study on women with severe hot flushes in the UK using soya supplementation amounting to 80 mg of isoflavones per day, produced a statistically significant reduction in symptoms.

As the average Asian diet delivers between 50 and 100 mg of isoflavones per day, it would seem reasonable not to exceed this dose. This matches the level that has been found to have a therapeutic effect in several clinical trials, and therefore seems a good compromise.

Let's compare how much saturated fat and isoflavones a typical Western diet delivers when compared to a soya-rich non-vegetarian diet, and a soya-rich vegetarian diet.

Typical Western menu using home-cooked ingredients

Menu One

Qty		S.F.	T.F.	Prot.	Carbo.	Fibre	Phyto.
	Breakfast						
50 g (2 oz)	Porridge oats	0.1	2.5	7	27	2.3	Tr
150 ml (1/4 pt)	Whole cow's milk	2.5	4.1	4	5.5	0	
	Lunch						
2 slices	White bread	0	0.18	4	24	0.15	Tr
2 rashers	Bacon	1.3	4	11.7	0	0	
1	Fried egg	2.4	6.4	5.4	0	0	
	Dinner						
100 g (4 oz)	Steak	8.4	17	22	0	0	
100 g (4 oz)	Chips	7	13	2.6	24	0	
75 g (3 oz)	Peas	0	0	4.1	11	1.7	

	Dessert					
100 g (4 oz)	Apple pie	4.7	17	3.4	61	0.6
75 ml (3 fl oz)	Double cream	12	2.5	6	7	0
	Snacks					
1 standard	Mars bar	7.6	11	5	17	0
100 g (4 oz)	Whole milk yogurt	1.7	2.5	6	7	0
Kcal		429	727	324	708	
Total calories	2233					

Expressed as a percentage of total calories

Saturated fat (S.F.)	19%
Total fat (T.F.)	33%
Protein	15%
Carbohydrates	32%
Phytoestrogens mg/day	Trace

Soya-rich non-vegetarian menu

Menu Two

Qty	Breakfast	S.F.	T.F.	Prot.	Carbo.	Fibre	Phyto.
50 g (2 oz)	Porridge oats	0.1	2.5	7	27	2.3	Tr
150 ml (¹/4 pt)	So Good soya milk	0.25	2.3	3.3	2	1.3	10 mg
25 g (1 oz)	Almonds*	0.7	5.1	3.4	12	1.7	
1 medium	Pear	0	0	0.7	25	2.3	
	Lunch						
2 slices	Wholemeal bread	0	2.0	6	28	3.2	Tr
50 g (2 oz)	Cheddar cheese	12	16.4	14	0	0	
100 g (4 oz)	Green salad	0	0	0.1	1	0.5	
1 medium	Apple*	0.1	0.5	0.3	21	1.06	
	Dinner						
100 g (4 oz)	Chicken and tofu burger	6.5	12.1	27.2	3.5	0.6	11 mg
1 medium	Jacket potato	0.1	0.2	4.7	51	1.2	
75 g (3 oz)	Green beans	0.1	0.2	1.2	5	1.1	
75 g (3 oz)	Sweetcorn	0.2	1.1	2.7	21	0.5	
	Dessert						
1 large	Stewed apple*	0.5	0.1	0.5	51	1.2	
75 ml (3 fl oz)	Soya Dream	0.75	8	1.5	1	0	13 mg
	Snacks						
100 g (4 oz)	Soya yogurt	0.6	3.6	5	3.9	0	12 mg
1	Bagel	0	2.6	11	56	0.22	
Kcal		207	510	351	1,218		
Total calories	2286						

Expressed as a percentage of total calories

Saturated Fat (S.F.)	9%
Total Fat (T.F.)	22%
Protein	15%
Carbohydrates	53%
Phytoestrogens mg/day	51 mg

* foods marked contain phytoestrogens, but there are no published figures so an additional 5 mg per day is allowed.

Soya-rich vegetarian menu

Menu Three

Qty		S.F.	T.F.	Prot.	Carbo.	Fibre	Phyto.
	Breakfast						
50 g (2 oz)	Porridge oats	0.1	2.5	7	27	2.3	Tr
150 ml (¹/4 pt)	So Good soya milk	0.25	2.3	3.3	2	1.3	10 mg
25 g (1 oz)	Almonds*	0.7	5.1	3.4	12	1.7	
1 medium	Apple*	0.1	0.5	0.3	21	1.06	
	Lunch						
75 g (3 oz)	Hummus	1.1	4.1	14	9	1.75	15 mg
1 slice	Rye bread	0	0.9	2.1	11	1.6	1 mg
100 g (4 oz)	Carrot and raisin salad	0.5	7.5	2.75	10.5	1.25	
	Dinner						
100 g (4 oz)	Indonesian tofu Kebabs with satay sauce	5	14	27.2	17.3	1.2	50 mg
100 g (4 oz)	Stir-fried mixed veg	1.6	3.6	3.9	19.5	3	
100 g (4 oz)	Basmati rice	0.1	0.4	4.8	45	0.21	Tr
	Dessert						
100 g (4 oz)	Soya yogurt	0.6	3.6	5	3.9	0	12 mg
	Snacks						
1 medium	Banana	0.2	0.6	1.2	27	0.57	
Kcal		92	405	300	829		
Total calories	1626						

Expressed as a percentage of total calories

Saturated Fat (S.F.)	5%
Total Fat (T.F.)	23%
Protein	18%
Carbohydrates	51%
Phytoestrogens mg/day	93 mg

* foods marked contain phytoestrogens, but there are no published figures so an additional 5 mg per day is allowed.

As you can see, by eating a more wholesome diet, you will be reducing your intake of saturated animal fat, while dramatically increasing your intake of those wonderful isoflavones. The wholesome, but non-vegetarian diet, still delivers over 50 mg of isoflavones per day, which is known to be sufficient to have a therapeutic effect. The vegetarian menu provides even more isoflavones, but you need not follow a strict vegetarian diet unless you want to. Further information about the amount of phytoestrogen required on a daily basis can be found in Part Two, Eating for Health – The Phyto Factor Diet.

What about men and children?

Asian men consume between 40 and 70 mg of isoflavones daily and have done so for centuries, without, it seems, any adverse health effects. In fact, you will see from Chapter 10, Phytoestrogens and Cancer Prevention, that scientists believe that far fewer Asian men die from prostate cancer because of their regular phytoestrogen intake. Like women, it appears that men can only benefit from the levels of phytoestrogens that are currently being suggested.

Asian children also consume phytoestrogens daily, once again without any adverse health reports. While I would not suggest that you go out of your way to feed children a phytoestrogen-rich diet, scientifically there seems no harm in them consuming soya products as part of a varied and nutritious diet. The same recommendation would apply to pregnant women. Asian women and vegetarians have happily been consuming a wide variety of vegetarian protein, including soya, for hundreds of years.

5

GOOD SOYA VS. NOT SO GOOD SOYA

The good news is that consuming soya products has tremendous health benefits, but the bad news is that not all soya foods these days are as Mother Nature intended. For approximately 60 per cent of *processed* foods in UK shops contain genetically-engineered soya beans, and there is currently no way of identifying which they are. GM crops are being introduced with minimal consultation with Parliament or the public despite the fact that the public doesn't want them. A 1998 MORI survey revealed that 61 per cent of people don't want to eat genetically modified crops and 77 per cent of people support a ban on the commercial growing of GM crops. The House of Commons can-teen avoids GM food, yet the government is happy for it to be sold on the supermarket shelves..

GENETIC ENGINEERING

The concept of genetic engineering is not new. Tomato products have been genetically adjusted for some time, by having the gene turned off that causes the tomato to ripen. Much of the tomato purée that sits on supermarket shelves has small print on its label informing us that it has been genetically modified. Were genetically engineered soya products labelled similarly, there would be no problem, as we would still be able to make a choice. However, the American Soya Bean Association, which is responsible for most of the world's soya crop, has failed to get its members to separate modified beans from unmodified beans, because of the cost. The giant American food company Monsanto is now churning out genetically modified soya beans by the ton, which turn up on our dinner plates without us even knowing. Once processed, these modified beans are indistinguishable from soya beans in their natural state and they are used in common foods including assorted pies, biscuits, cooking oils, margarine and pasta, and many more besides.

Processed products

Full fat soya flour	Soya lecithin	Soya oil	De-fatted soya flour	Soya concentrate	Soya isolate
Breads	Bakery products	Battered/ breaded snacks and vegetables	Baked goods	Meat products	Cheeses
Doughnut mixes	Confectionery		Pie crusts	Protein drinks	Coffee whiteners
Instant milk drinks	Chocolate coatings	Breads		Soup bases	Frozen desserts
Pancake flours	Ice creams	Cooking oils		Gravies	Infant formulas
Pie crusts	Margarines	Crackers			Meat products
	Shortenings	Frozen fried seafood			Soya milk
	Medicines	Margarines			
	Vitamins	Mayonnaises			
		Non-dairy creamers			
		Potato & corn chips			
		Salad dressings			
		Sauces			
		Shortenings			
		Soups			
		Stocks/bases			
		Taco shells			
		Whipped toppings			

(Adapted from information provided by Monsanto)

WHAT DOES GENETIC ENGINEERING INVOLVE?

Every cell in an organism, whether bacterium, plant, animal or human, contains a complete set of genes, known as the genome. The genome of a human cell contains 23 pairs of chromosomes which are located within the nucleus of each cell, and each chromosome consists of two very long deoxyribonucleic acid (DNA) molecules, folded together in a double helix or spiral shape. The genes are separated from each other by DNA, which does not form part of the gene. In genetic engineering, an organism's DNA is reorganised or removed, or indeed added to, and the result is that specific characteristics are modified. In the case of genetically modified soya beans, Monsanto introduced a gene from a bacterium into soya beans to produce a variety resistant to being sprayed with the company's herbicide, Roundup. When Roundup is sprayed on the soya bean plant fields after the plants have been modified, only the weeds will die. Very ingenious.

Is it safe to consume genetically modified food?

There are varying opinions about the possible risks and benefits associated with consuming genetically engineered food, but it is fair to say that most of those who are in favour have commercial connections somewhere along the line. The main worry is that genetically engineered food has not been thoroughly tested for long-term effects on animals, let alone people, and there seems to be no requirement for the long-term effects to be monitored. When soya is modified to make it resistant to an all-purpose weedkiller herbicide, there is a risk that the plant could contain higher levels of residues, which, in turn could worsen allergies in some and cause skin problems in others. The Monsanto Roundup soya bean has been declared safe to eat by the American and European regulatory bodies, but concerned nutritionists argue that food gene technology is still so new that the long-term risks are not yet quantifiable. Much of the justification advanced for genetically engineered food products is the widely aired claim that genetically engineered foods will '*feed the world*'.

Swiss researchers have discovered that maize spliced with a gene toxic to cornborers, an agricultural pest, proved lethal to the green lacewing, a beneficial insect that normally preys on the pests. In October 1977 *The Times* newspaper reported that Dundee ladybirds which ate aphids fed on genetically modified potatoes laid fewer eggs and only lived half as long as normal, which is a bit worrying to say the least.

Equally concerning is that Monsanto seemed to have cornered the market in a major way. They have promoted sales of their genetically engineered Roundup Ready soya beans by getting farmers to sign contracts that prevent them saving, selling or giving away seeds or any material 'derived therefrom'. The contract obliges them to use Monsanto herbicides and give Monsanto monitoring access to their farms for three years! I happened to catch an interview on the BBC with a group of US farmers who had been invited to sell their wares in the UK, where fortunately there is still a demand for unmodified soya beans.

A problem foreseen by critics of genetically engineered food is the transfer of allergenic potential along with the transfer of genes from one organism to another. In other words, people start getting allergies to things they never used to have problems with because of GE.

Blood serum from people known to be allergic to Brazil nuts was tested for the appropriate antibody response to the gene transferred to the soya bean. Seven out of nine volunteers did show such a response to the GE soya bean and the researchers concluded that the allergenicity had been transferred with the transferred gene.

Consumers' rights

Greenpeace and other organisations, including FLAG and the Genetics Forum in the UK and the Australian Consumers' Association, are actively calling for new labelling laws which will identify the 'gene bean'. The Australian Consumers' Association has, it seems, convinced the Federal Government that it should label foods that contain genetically modified food, but no law has been passed as yet. The absence of legislation is obviously a violation of our rights that must be resolved. If you would like to add your support to the ongoing campaigns, you will find the addresses of the campaigning associations in the Useful Addresses list, which begins on page 259. Science funding is becoming more biased towards genetic engineering ahead of other approaches. In the UK there is now the Biotechnology and Biological Sciences Research Council where once we had the Agriculture and Food Research Council.

As well as public protests, some manufacturers and major retailers have refused to stock products containing genetically modified soya or maize. Instead they are actively seeking an alternative supply, and demanding segregation of the genetically modified beans from the rest of the crop. Fifty per cent of consumers surveyed in Australia definitely stated that they wanted genetically modified products clearly labelled. Surely, we all have the right to choose what we consume?

Labelling

Until food producers are required by law to state on the label that their products have been genetically modified, we the consumers have to pick our way through the confusion. European law on the labelling of GM foods, known as the Novel Food Regulations, was introduced in May 1997. This legislation stated that GM foods or ingredients did not have to be labelled if they were more or less identical or 'substantially equivalent' to ordinary foods and ingredients. The concept of substantial equivalence has never been properly defined, but what it really means is that if a GM food can be characterised as substantially equivalent to its 'natural' derivative, it can be assumed to pose no new health risks and hence is acceptable for commercial use. This rule is somewhat vague, and it is this vagueness that makes the concept useful to industry but unacceptable to the consumer.

The Novel Foods Regulations meant that manufacturers and supermarkets had to label their products only if GM foods or ingredients:

- were nutritionally or compositionally different
- contained material that might affect health, such as by triggering allergies
- raised ethical issues, e.g. animal genes in plant foods for vegetarians.

Public pressure led to new labelling rules in 1998, which were agreed for the whole of the European Union. These stated that food and ingredients derived from GM soya and maize, and which contained 'detectable levels' of GM material, had to be labelled as 'produced from genetically modified soya/maize.' Detectable levels means that traces of protein or DNA are present in the final product. The more refined a product is, the fewer traces of genetically modified ingredients; therefore the consumer could be eating derivatives from GM products whithout knowing it. In effect, this meant that the vast majority of additives and flavourings derived from GM soya and maize did not need to be labelled. Furthermore, processing aids, such as enzymes produced using gene technology, were excluded from these labelling regulations.

The Food and Drugs Administration announced in 1999 that it would review its policies on genetically modified crops, including whether to label food containing genetically modified ingredients. The US Food Safety Administration does not require products to be labelled, on the grounds that genetically modified crops are essentially the same as traditional varieties and therefore pose no health risk!

The EC proposal to allow foods to be labelled as GM free if they contain no more than 1 per cent of genetically modified derivatives was passed in Brussels on 22 October 1999. This agreement meant that food contaminated with 1 per cent or less of a GM ingredient would escape the gene-modified labelling regime. This caused tremendous outrage among green groups, who were angry at the final decision. However, there was another argument in favour of the agreement. Without it, small companies doing their utmost to source non-GM suppliers would have been penalised, because they might not have had the money or the resources to achieve such 'unrealistic' goals.

A number of food manufacturers and retailers have told Friends of the Earth that they are operating to much lower contamination thresholds than those agreed by the European Commission. Friends of the

Earth believes that the best way of securing GM-free ingredients is a properly audited system of documentation and segregation of all GM crops and derivatives from farm to plate.

An interim rule we have adopted at the Women's Nutritional Advisory Service (WNAS), is that most wholefood and soya food companies are using soya beans that have not been tampered with, and their soya products are therefore safe to buy. However, we have rightly or wrongly assumed that most processed food with soya included on the contents list is likely to be the genetically engineered variety.

In 1998 the WNAS carried out a survey to determine which manufacturers used GM foods and ingredients and those that didn't. Because the GMO scene is rapidly changing, and many food retailers were in the transitional stages of phasing out their GM stocks whilst trying to source new supplies, it presented us with the difficult task of deciding in which category to place them, i.e. those who use/don't use GMOs. We therefore felt it appropriate not to publish the results of the survey. Within one year of conducting the first survey, we have seen an encouraging trend in response to genetic engineering from the major food manufacturers and retailers. The general consensus now is that the main food manufacturers and supermarkets have either withdrawn all genetically engineered foods or are in the transitional stages of removing them.

6

OTHER ESSENTIAL NUTRITION

As well as being rich in phytoestrogens, an optimum diet needs to fulfil a number of other important criteria, as research quite clearly shows that diet influences health prospects and, to a large extent, the length of our lives. The major causes of death in developed countries are heart disease and cancer, which are influenced to a large degree by dietary and environmental factors. Up to 50 per cent of people with heart disease or cancer could probably have prevented or delayed the onset of their illness if they had eaten a better diet (or stopped smoking). This is particularly important for those who become ill at a relatively young age, i.e. before 65 years. Furthermore, many minor illnesses are also influenced by diet and these include problems such as migraine headaches, high blood pressure, arthritis, kidney stones, premenstrual syndrome, eczema, fatigue, irritable bowel syndrome, insomnia and anxiety, and these just represent the tip of the iceberg.

When we are children our parents teach us how to eat, dress, wash and generally look after ourselves and we are taught at school how to read, write and add up. But where and how do we learn about our bodies' requirements? It is not at school, neither is it at evening classes, as they seem to concentrate there on car maintenance and the secrets of computer mechanics. The woman, who is often regarded as the 'nutritional head of the household', and is expected to meet the demands of her family's nutrient needs as well as her own, has little or no training for this job. When considered rationally, this seems outrageous, especially as we trade in both our cars and our computers from time to time, but only have one body to last a lifetime.

WHAT IS A BALANCED DIET?

Because we are so often told by doctors that a balanced diet is all that we need to maintain our health, the WNAS conducted a random survey a few years ago to find out what people understood by the term 'a balanced diet'. We also asked which foods contained key vitamins like A, B, C, D and E, and some key minerals like calcium, magnesium, zinc and iron. The negative results of this survey would have been entertaining were it not for the fact that the consequences of an unbalanced diet may severely affect the quality of human health. The only information that people seemed to have about their diet were the basic lessons from school, if they could remember them. Apart from knowing facts such as 'oranges contain vitamin C' and 'liver contains iron', hardly anyone had a clue as to what actually constituted a sound balanced diet, or how much of each nutrient was required each day for their body size (or anyone else's body size for that matter).

Although magazine articles are among the main sources of information about diet, confusion abounds as we lurch from one diet scandal to another. First we hear that alcohol is bad for us and that animal fats will cause our cholesterol levels to rise. Then we hear that we should be drinking two or three glasses of wine each day to prevent heart disease, and that fats have little influence on our cholesterol levels. Should we be eating liver regularly, or does it contain too much vitamin A? Will soft cheeses and uncooked eggs give us listeria and salmonella? Is decaffeinated tea and coffee *really* better for us or will the other methylxanthines get us anyway? We could well be forgiven for putting our heads in the sand and hoping for the best. Trying to sort out the dietary myths from the facts is an arduous task for anyone.

ESSENTIAL NUTRIENTS

In order to understand fully the role of vitamins and minerals in health, it is necessary to have some idea about the part that each nutrient has to play. A truly balanced diet must provide an adequate supply of energy and protein, plus essential vitamins, minerals and specialised fats called essential fatty acids. The majority of energy comes from fats and carbohydrates in the diet, and a small amount from protein-rich foods.

Proteins, fats, carbohydrates and fibre are all essential for normal body function. Let's look briefly at the function they serve.

PROTEIN

This term is used to describe a series of complex chemicals that are widely found in many nutritious foods. Proteins are made up of amino acids, the essential building blocks, as well as many hormones, enzymes and other agents involved in the intricate metabolism of living organisms. If protein intake is not adequate in the diet, then tissue growth and repair cannot take place, and protein-rich tissues break down, especially muscle.

48

Sources of protein

Protein can be found in both animal and vegetarian sources – meat, eggs, dairy products including milk and cheese, peas, beans, soya products, lentils, nuts, seeds and, to a very small extent, rice and potatoes. It is wise to have a wide variety of protein sources in your diet, especially if you are a vegetarian.

FATS

Fats provide us with energy. There is a variety of different fats, which are all chemically similar, and per gram weight they provide us with over twice the energy content of carbohydrate or sugar (9 calories per gram compared to 3.75 calories per gram carbohydrate).

Animal fats

The majority of animal fats are saturated and serve only as a source of calories. Saturated fats are not essential and have a chemical structure of a chain of carbon atoms saturated with hydrogen. This means that they are usually solid at room temperature. A diet rich in these saturated animal fats, and lacking in fibre, vitamins and minerals will often predispose to heart disease (see Chapter 11, Phytoestrogens reduce heart disease).

Vegetable fats

Many, but not all, vegetable fats are polyunsaturates and these include the specialised essential fatty acids (EFAs), which are used in the building structure of cells, especially those of the skin and nervous system, as well as being a source of calories. They are called essential as they cannot be made by the body but instead need to come from the diet. Chemically these fats or oils are unsaturated and are able to accept more hydrogen molecules. This means that they are usually liquid at room temperature. Olive oil and rapeseed oil are rich in mono-unsaturates, which are not essential, but they do not add to the risk of heart disease in the way that saturated fats do. Good sources of the essential fatty acids are corn, sunflower and safflower oils which provide the omega-6 series of EFAs. Oily fish such as mackerel, herring and salmon, soya bean and walnut oil and to a small extent rapeseed oil, linseed and linseed oil provide the omega-3 series.

Omega-3 essential fatty acids

These are unsaturated fats that play a major role in the control of inflammation. They help to control cholesterol levels and maintain our cardiovascular health, and the health of our immune system, our liver and the nervous system. Rich sources are oily fish including mackerel, herring, salmon, pilchards and sardines, plus linseeds, walnuts, rapeseed and soya products.

CARBOHYDRATES

The term 'carbohydrates' is a collective term for the different sugars and starches in our diet. Starches are composed of many individual sugar molecules, predominantly glucose, and are broken down by the digestive system into these simple sugars, some of which are better for us than others. The simple sugars are glucose, fructose and galactose, which is part of the sugar found in milk. Table sugar, which is also called sucrose, is made up of one glucose and one fructose unit joined together. Its commercial production from sugar cane and sugar beet leads to the complete loss of vitamins and minerals found in these parent sources. A similar refining process to prepare white flour from wholemeal flour leads to a substantial reduction in essential vitamins and minerals. Sugars and starch-rich foods all require vitamin B and magnesium in order to be metabolised. Sucrose, and to a lesser extent fructose, also predispose to tooth decay.

Sources of refined carbohydrates

Cakes, biscuits, sweets, chocolate, table sugar, white bread, white pasta and many breakfast cereals are all refined products that have been depleted of many essential nutrients. Fortunately white flour and some breakfast cereals are fortified with vitamins, and flour has added calcium; this helps to make up for these nutritional losses.

Nutritious carbohydrate sources

All cereals, potatoes, rice and root vegetables and pulses are sources of nutritious carbohydrates. Fresh fruits and vegetables also provide a mixture of sugars – mainly fructose and a small amount of starch.

FIBRE

Fibre is a type of carbohydrate that comes from the cell wall of plants, cellulose, and remains undigested in the gut. Because of its water-retaining properties, it forms the bulk of our stool. There are many types of fibre with differing properties. Most of us associate fibre-rich foods with those containing bran, for example, but bran may inhibit the absorption of certain essential nutrients. Fibre from fruit, vegetables, soya products and oats, however, not only provides us with a supply of good nutrients, but also helps to reduce cholesterol levels by binding with the cholesterol before being excreted in the faeces.

Good sources of fibre

A diet rich in fruit, vegetables, salad and cereals, linseeds and soya products lowers blood cholesterol and the risk of heart disease, as well as providing many essential vitamins and minerals.

VITAMINS AND MINERALS

There are some 15 vitamins, 15 minerals, and eight to ten amino acids that have been isolated as being essential for normal body function. These nutrients are synergistic, which means they rely on each other in order to keep the body functioning at an optimum level. If you liken the body to a computer for a moment, the computer can only function when it has the correct data and commands fed into it; otherwise it refuses to work or breaks down altogether. Similarly, our bodies require the correct input of nutrients. When one or more nutrients is in short supply the body cannot function properly, and symptoms, be they physical or mental, occur.

Although it is true that severe nutritional deficiencies are rare in countries like the UK, Australia, New Zealand and the USA, poor intakes of a number of nutrients are acknowledged in some 20 per cent of women of child-bearing age. Combined nutritional inadequacies are likely to have an adverse affect on hormone function and on health in general during the ageing process.

NUTRITIONAL NEEDS THROUGH THE AGES

Our bodies are indeed very complex machines that have very specific requirements in order that they may function efficiently. Women particularly have varying needs, not just during their years of physical growth and development, but through each phase as it presents itself. The nutritional requirements for pregnancy are quite different, for example, from those of a woman at the time of the menopause.

To understand your own nutrient needs better, you need a little knowledge about each individual nutrient and the signs and symptoms of deficiency. The following chart will give you some idea about the changing needs throughout life.

Understanding your nutrient needs

Nutrient	Food sources	What they do	Who is at risk	Symptoms	Visible signs
Vitamin A	*Retinol (animal vitamin A)* Liver, all dairy products and margarine *Beta carotene (vegetable vitamin A)* All yellow, green, and orange fruits and vegetables	Essential for vision, especially in the dark, for growth and resistance to infection	The ill, elderly and poorly fed pre-school children	Poor night vision, recurrent chest infections	None
Vitamin B1 (Thiamine)	Meat, fish, nuts, whole-grains and fortified breakfast cereals	Essential in the metabolism of sugar, especially in nerves and muscles	Alcohol consumers, women on the pill, breast-feeding mothers, high consumers of sugar	Depression, anxiety, poor appetite, nausea, personality change	None usually! Heart, nerve and muscle problems if severe
Vitamin B2 (Riboflavin)	Milk, meats, fish and vegetables	Involved in energy release from fats and carbohydrates	Those on a poor diet	Deficiency, rarely severe	Mild fatigue and possibly burning feet Peeling of the skin on the lips Red ring around the iris of the eye
Potassium	All vegetables and fruit	Needed for the health of all cells, especially muscles and the nervous system	The elderly, after prolonged vomiting, with use of some diuretics and poor diet	Weakness, low blood pressure and muscle cramps	None
Selenium	Most wholesome foods, especially seafoods	Involved in two enzymes that protect inflamed and damaged tissues and help thyroid function	The ill elderly, those on a very poor diet, possibly those with heart failure, alcoholics and long-standing mal-absorption	None that are specific, just not well	None

Nutrient	Food sources	What they do	Who is at risk	Symptoms	Visible signs
Chromium	All wholesome foods, not sugar and other refined carbohydrates	Helps in the action of insulin Deficiency causes a diabetic-like state	The elderly, life-long consumers of junk food!	Those of diabetes or of a low blood sugar with episodic weakness and sugar craving	Perhaps a large waistline or sweet wrappers in their pockets!
Essential fatty acids omega-3	Cod liver oil, mackerel, herring	Help control inflammation	Those on a poor diet	None	None
Fish and related oils	Salmon, canola and soya bean oil	Reduce calcium losses in urine	Older people, diabetics, drinkers	None	None
Essential fatty acids omega-6, evening primrose and related oils	Sunflower, safflower and corn oils, many nuts (not peanuts) and seeds, green vegetables	Control of inflammation, needed for health of nervous system, skin and blood vessels	Those on a poor diet, diabetics and drinkers. Also those with severe eczema and premenstrual breast tenderness	None	Possibly dry skin
Folic acid	All green leafy vegetables, liver and fortified cereals	Help maintain the health of the nervous system and the blood	Those on a poor diet, those taking anti-epileptic medication, coeliacs, and a percentage of the normal population of child-bearing women who are at increased risk of having a child with a neural tube defect	Often none Possibly depression, fatigue and poor memory	None unless anaemic
Iron	Meat, wholegrains, nuts, eggs and fortified breakfast cereals	Essential to make blood haemoglobin Many other tissues need iron for energy reactions	Women who have heavy periods (e.g. coil users), vegetarians, especially if tea or coffee drinkers, women with recurrent thrush	Fatigue, poor energy, depression, poor digestion, sore tongue, cracking at corners of mouth	Pale complexion, brittle nails, cracking at corners of mouth

Nutrient	Food sources	What they do	Who is at risk	Symptoms	Visible signs
Zinc	Meat, wholegrains, nuts, peas, beans, lentils	Essential for normal growth, mental function, hormone production and resistance to infection	Vegetarians, especially tea and coffee drinkers, alcohol consumers, long-term users of diuretics (water pills)	Poor mental function, skin problems in general, repeated infections	Eczema, acne, greasy or dry facial skin
Magnesium	Green vegetables, wholegrains, ·Brazil and almond nuts, many other non-junk foods	Essential for sugar and energy metabolism, needed for healthy nerves and muscles	Women with PMS! (some 50 per cent may be lacking), long-term diuretic users, alcohol consumers	Nausea, apathy, loss of appetite, depression	
Calcium	Milk, cheese, bread, especially white, sardines, other fish with bones, green vegetables and beans	Needed for strong teeth and bones, also for normal nerve and muscle function Lack leads to osteoporosis – bone thinning	Low dairy consumers, heavy drinkers, smokers, women with early menopause Lack of exercise increases the rate of bone loss-calcium in later years	Usually none until osteoporotic fracture of hip or spine	Back pain, loss of height

7

PHYTOESTROGEN-RICH FOODS

THE A–Z OF SOYA FOODS

Beans

The soya beans we use today are closely related to those beans that first grew in ancient China. The soya bean plant is roughly hip-high, and the beans themselves grow in green pods, usually with two or three beans to a pod. The beans are often harvested when they are mature or dry, often yellow in colour, although in Asian countries they are sometimes harvested when they are well developed, but still green. Black and brown varieties are also grown, but these are less common. Soya beans can be consumed either fresh or dried. The soya beans intended for use as a fresh dish are harvested early and usually used in Asian countries, where they are served as a vegetable or a snack.

The preparation for fresh soya beans is simple, the pods are boiled in a pan for approximately 15 minutes, and the beans are removed from the pods before serving. An alternative method of preparing fresh soya beans is to remove them from the pod before cooking, and then simmer them for about 20 minutes, in a similar way to other vegetables. When they are tender, but crisp, they are ready to serve. They can be added to stir-fry dishes, be served as an hors d'oeuvre, or as a side dish. Outside Asia, fresh soya beans may not be so easy to find, although Asian supermarkets often sell them. If you grow your own vegetables you could include soya beans in your selection and expect a reasonable crop of fresh beans during the summer months.

Like most other legumes, over time soya beans lose their green colour as they ripen and harden. They have a long shelf life in their mature state, but do need to be soaked in water, preferably overnight, prior to being cooked, as they require re-hydrating. Even after being soaked, they still need thorough cooking for approximately three hours, and the cooking water should be discarded. Once the bean is easily crushable between your fingers, it is ready to serve.

Cooked soya beans have what is often described as a 'beany' flavour, which is stronger than the taste of most other beans. There are a variety of ways to serve them including soups, casseroles, stews, curries and burgers. Soya beans alone have a fairly bland flavour, but can be enhanced with the addition of herbs or spices during the cooking process. If you are planning to add tomatoes to the dish, it is best to add them towards the end of the cooking time, as they can make the soya beans tough.

Breads

As the benefits of soya are becoming known, some food manufacturers are beginning to include soya flour and linseeds into bread recipes. Examples of these are the Burgen Loaf in the UK, the Burgen Soya-Lin Loaf available in Australia, and Country Fare Soya and Linseed Bread in New Zealand. The availability of these new loaves makes it easier for those consuming a Western diet to include soya and linseeds into their diet on a regular basis. Studies have shown that just by adding the equivalent of four slices of soya and linseed bread into the diet each day it is possible to reduce menopausal hot flushes by 40 per cent. It is also possible to make home-made bread using a combination of soya flour and other flours. On pages 240–245 you will find some of our successful bread recipes using soya flour and in some cases linseeds. I purchased a bread maker fairly recently, which has proved to be a tremendous investment. I simply place the ingredients in the machine and return three hours later to remove a fresh loaf, and the smell that wafts through the house while it is cooking is amazing.

Cereals

Brands of muesli containing soya flakes and grits are also available in the healthfood shops, and equally home-made varieties can be concocted (see our recipes on page 183). Soya-based muesli can also be added to biscuits, muffins or cake mixture.

Cheese

Soya cheese is the product of soya milk, in the same way that cheese is the product of dairy milk. It can be used in sandwiches, or grated or sprinkled onto dishes like bakes, pastas or pizza, and even used in sauces. In my experience it doesn't toast very well.

Cream

Soya Dream produced by Provamel could be mistaken for single cream. It is a lactose, dairy and gluten-free alternative to cream, and, like cream, can be used in cooking, in coffee or poured over fruit. Recipes using soya cream are included in Chapter 19.

Drinks

Soya drinks, which are a variation of soya milk, come in the form of milk-shakes and smoothies. There are many commercial varieties available, and in addition they can be whipped up in the blender at home. See pages 247–249 for some suggestions.

Flakes

Soya flakes are made from toasted, dried soya beans, which are then split and rolled into flakes. They can be added to a wide variety of dishes including breads, muffins, cereals, biscuits, crumbles and even savoury dishes like meatballs and bakes.

Flour

Soya flour is made from mature soya beans that have been roasted, rolled into flakes and ground into a powder that can be used in baking. It has a 50 per cent protein content, but as it does not contain gluten in the same way as other flours, it cannot be used as a complete substitute in bread recipes as it prevents the yeast from rising. It also tends to be heavier than many other flours. In bread recipes, we tend to use approximately one part soya flour, one part rice flour and one part corn or potato flour. It can also be used in muffins, pancakes, biscuits and cakes. It adds protein to dishes, moisture and a nutty flavour, so is often favoured by vegetarians. Both full fat and 'de-fatted' versions, where the oil has been extracted during the processing, are available. When used in a mixture for fried products (e.g. pakora), it tends to reduce the absorption of oil far more than other flours. It should be stored in a cool, dry place in an airtight container to prevent it from going rancid.

Grits

These are made from mature, dried soya beans that have been lightly toasted and then cracked into small pieces. Grits maintain the flavour and the nutritional value of the soya bean, but they have a fairly high fat content, so once again should be stored in a cool, dry place in an airtight container. They cook more quickly than soya beans, within approximately 45 minutes, without needing to be pre-soaked. They should be cooked in a similar way to rice, with three parts water to one part grits. Once they have been brought to the boil, they should be simmered until all the water has been absorbed. They can be mixed with other grains to add protein, or added to stews, burgers or pasta sauces as their texture is similar to minced beef.

Lecithin

This is a by-product of soya oil, which is a natural emulsifier and lubricant. If you read labels carefully, you will see that it is widely used in pre-prepared foods ranging from chocolate bars to savoury foods. It has a reputation as a cholesterol-lowering agent, and is also available in capsule and granule form from healthfood shops.

Meats

Soya is a well known meat substitute, and can be made to look, smell and almost taste like the real thing. There is practically no end to the variety of impersonating roles that soya takes on. For example it is used in vegetarian burgers, sausages, bacon, patties, nuggets, hot dogs and mince. These days soya 'meat' products can often be found in the supermarkets as well as the healthfood stores. It is usually available in frozen, canned or dried varieties, which can be grilled, baked, barbecued or pan-fried, as well as being used as a substitute in meat recipes. Although it is a rich source of protein, and is lower in fat and cholesterol than real meat, unlike meat it is a poor source of vitamin B12 unless it has been fortified with vitamins and minerals. Compared to many other soya products soya 'meat' often has a low content of isoflavones.

Milk

Like dairy milk, soya milk is a versatile liquid that can be consumed as a drink, or used in milk shakes, sauces, soups, cereals or in cooking in place of cow's milk. In years gone by it had a reputation for having a beany flavour, but with improved processing techniques most products now have a very light and acceptable flavour. The So Good range seems to have a particularly acceptable flavour. It is made from soya protein isolate, the protein portion of the soya bean in an almost pure form, which perhaps explains why it does not have the traditional beany flavour often associated with soya beverages. The isolate is extracted from the soya flour in a process that involves subjecting the flour firstly to acidic and then alkaline conditions to remove excess carbohydrates and fats.

By using soya protein isolate, So Good has managed to provide a very acceptable cow's milk replacement, with about the same calcium content. Soya milk is lactose free and can therefore be used by those intolerant to lactose, and by vegans. Although it does not inherently contain as much vitamin D, calcium or vitamin B12 as cow's milk, many commercial products are fortified with these. So Good, for example, is fortified with the minerals calcium, magnesium, potassium and phosphorus, in amounts similar to those found in milk. So Good also contains vitamin C, vitamins B1, B2, B3 and B12, and vitamin A. As well as being sold as plain milk, flavoured varieties are often available, including chocolate, strawberry, mocha and vanilla. So Good has also introduced So Good Lite, which is a reduced fat product. In the West, soya milk can be found both in supermarkets and in healthfood shops, whereas in Asian countries it is sold by street vendors or even delivered to the doorstep. It usually comes in long-life containers that do not need refrigerating until the carton has been opened. It can be consumed as a hot or cold beverage, used in tea, coffee or substitutes, or used as the base for a fruit shake. The recipe section which begins on page 179 contains many recipes that include So Good, particularly in soups, breads, and fruit shakes.

Miso

Miso is a fermented soya bean paste made by mixing soya beans, salt, water and rice or barley. It is then stored in cedar vats and left to ferment for up to three years. 'Quick' miso is also available, which is aged for only a few days and helped along by chemicals and pasteurisation, but it has an inferior taste.

Miso has a distincive, full-bodied flavour and is an essential condiment in any Chinese or Japanese kitchen. Many Japanese start their day with a bowl of miso soup; it is packed with protein and a very rich source of isoflavones. However, it has an exceedingly high sodium (salt) content and should be avoided by anyone who has high blood pressure, or who is on a restricted salt diet for other health reasons. It is thought that a diet rich in salt may contribute to stomach cancer, but equally, miso is thought to help rid the body of radiation (see page 106). Most miso available in the West has a smooth texture, similar to that of peanut butter, whereas in Asian countries a chunky variety is also available. Since traditional miso is unpasteurised it should be stored in the refrigerator, where it can sit for up to one year. The white mould that appears can be scraped off and used in cooking, as it is simply an extension of the fermentation process. As it has such a salty flavour it only needs to be used in small quantities. One quarter of a cup of miso should be mixed with a litre of water to make a soup stock. It is also wonderful in marinades, spreads and sauces.

Natto

This is another fermented soya product traditionally made by incubating whole cooked soya beans in straw. These days natto is produced commercially by fermenting the cooked soya beans with *Bacillus natto*, and incubating the mixture in plastic bags until it develops a sticky coat. This process gives it its cheese-like texture and pungent smell. It is used by the Japanese in cooking, soups and for spreads. It is an excellent source of both protein and isoflavones, and a rich source of fibre.

Oil

Although soya bean oil does not contain isoflavones, as it is now a widely used vegetable oil it is worth concentrating on some of its other health properties. Unlike the majority of vegetable oils, soya oil is a rich source of omega-3 and omega-6 fatty acids, similar to that found in marine fish oils. Chapter 11 on heart disease talks about the benefits of these essential fatty acids, and their ability to lower both blood cholesterol and blood pressure and to inhibit the formation of blood clots. Soya oil also contains linoleic acid, which may help to prevent certain forms of cancer. It is derived from soya beans during the processing and is commonly found in commercially prepared foods and salad dressings. It is ideally suited for stir-fries, and can be used in home-made dressings. However, as with any oil, it should be used sparingly, remembering that we need to keep our total fat intake to no more than 20 per cent of our total calorie intake.

Okara

This product is made from the pulp of the soya bean, which remains when the liquid has been squeezed out. It inevitably contains the most fibrous part of the bean, including the hulls. It can be used in soups, added to salads, or used in muffins, biscuits and croquettes. It has a light fluffy texture and absorbs flavours well. Alternatively, it can be used to replace other grains when cooking. It does have a relatively short shelf life, so it needs to be refrigerated and consumed within a few days. Studies have shown that okara is an excellent cholesterol-lowering agent. It is also a rich source of protein and isoflavones.

Pasta

Soya flour is now being used in some brands of pasta such as Soyaroni, and Orgran soya and rice pasta and gluten-free pasta such as wheat-free lasagne sheets. These pastas can be used in soups, casseroles, or combined with your favourite sauces and Parmesan cheese.

Protein isolate

A protein-rich powder, known as soya protein isolate, is sold in health-food shops. Studies have shown that it has a valuable role in helping to lower cholesterol levels, see Chapter 11 on phytoestrogens and heart disease on page 111. It has higher protein levels than soya flour, usually in excess of 90 per cent, and is both fat and carbohydrate free. Because of the concentration of soya protein, it is an excellent source of isoflavones. Produced commercially with the intention of it being mixed into a drink, it does have other uses: as a non-dairy creamer, a meat extender to reduce levels of animal fat in products like burgers and it can also be found in weight-loss and muscle-building drinks and in meal-replacement bars. Protein isolate can be used in home baking, sprinkled on to cereals and fruit, or added to the ingredients in the blender.

Roasted soya nuts

Soya nuts have been accepted into the Western diet as a pre-dinner snack as they resemble peanuts and can be found alongside peanuts in many supermarkets and healthfood shops. They are a product of soya beans, which have been deep fried or roasted. They can easily be prepared at home, by pre-soaking mature soya beans for three hours, then roasting them on a greased sheet until they are golden brown and crispy. They can be salted if required and stored in an airtight container. Use them for snacks or add them to biscuits, cakes or to the cooking. They are a rich source of isoflavones, plus protein and fibre, but like nuts are also a rich source of calories.

Sauce

Soya sauce, one of the most popular condiments in the world, is another fermented product of the soya bean. The traditional soya sauce is known as 'shoyu' or 'tamari', and is quite different from the commercial soya sauce that is widely available in supermarkets, which is made from defatted soya bean meal and wheat which is mixed with a combination of chemicals, caramel, corn syrup and flavouring. Shoyu is made by combining roasted soya beans, wheat and *Aspergillus* mould, which develops into a culture known as 'koji'. After three days this is mixed with salt water and brewed in fermentation tanks for up to 18 months, after which it is further refined and pasteurised. The flavour of the two sauces is quite different.

Shoyu and tamari are available in almost all healthfood shops and some supermarkets. Like miso, soya sauce has an extremely salty flavour, and should be consumed in moderation and avoided by those who have a predisposition to high blood pressure or require a low-salt diet.

Snacks

As well as soya nuts and chips, we are now seeing some delicious soya-containing snack bars entering the market. The manufacturers of

Wallaby bars, those great favourites of mine when I visit Australia, are now producing rice, fruit and nut bars enriched with soya and calcium and exporting them to New Zealand and the UK. These are nutritious and can be carried around in your bag for an in-between meal snack instead of a bar of chocolate! It is possible to bake snack bars which include soya, linseeds and other goodies and they freeze well too. See pages 235–240 for examples of our experiments.

Sprouts

Soya beans can be sprouted in the same way as other beans. They take between five and ten days to sprout, and end up resembling a mung bean. Very popular in Chinese cooking, as well as being a good source of isoflavones they are a good source of protein and fibre and have a particularly high vitamin C content. They are great in stir-fries and bakes and additionally can be added to salads.

Tempeh

Tempeh is an Indonesian speciality that has been consumed for over 2,000 years. It is so popular in Indonesia that it is sold on the streets as a delicacy, wrapped in banana leaves, or on skewers. In recent years it has become a popular vegetarian dish in Western countries, and can be found on menus of vegetarian restaurants and in health-food stores. It is a fermented soya bean patty, which is traditionally prepared in Indonesian households. Tempeh is made from soya beans that are soaked overnight, and then cooked until soft. Powder of the mould *Rhizopus oryzae*, or a piece of tempeh from the previous batch are then added as a starter, and the mixture is left to ferment for a further 24 hours. The flavour of tempeh is likened to strong mush-rooms, with a mildly nutty, smoky flavour. Its texture is chewy, which makes it an acceptable substitute for meat. It can be marinated, grilled, fried, steamed, grated, used in doner kebabs, chillies, stews, stir-fries or burgers, and even chopped into salads as mock chicken or combined with mayonnaise and vegetables like onions, peppers and celery and used as a sandwich filling. It is often sold frozen, and can be stored for a maximum of ten days in the refrigerator, and three months in the freezer. If you are able to purchase fresh tempeh it should have white flecks as opposed to black flecks, which indicate that it is stale. Tempeh is a rich source of isoflavones, fibre, protein, and the great thing about tempeh is that, unlike all other soya products, it is a good source of vitamin B12, usually only found in animal protein.

Toasted soya powder

This is made by grinding toasted soya beans into a fine powder. It is consumed in a variety of unusual ways around the world. In the Philippines it is used as a coffee substitute, whereas in China it is mixed with sugar and fat and used as a pastry filling. It is a product of soya that is not currently widely used in the West, but certainly one that we are now experimenting with in our cooking.

Textured vegetarian protein

This is often referred to as TVP, or TSP, textured soya protein, and is used widely by vegetarians and Asians as a meat substitute. It is made from defatted soya flour that is compressed until the protein fibres change in structure. When dry it has a granular appearance, but in order to be consumed it needs to be rehydrated, after which it takes on the appearance of minced beef, or even chunks of beef that are commonly used in stews or stir-fries. The rehydrating process for the 'mince' simply requires slightly less than one cup of boiling water to be poured over one cup of TVP. The chunks need to be covered in boiling water and simmered for a few minutes. It is also used as a chicken replacement, and it can replace meat in vegetarian meat loaves and pies. It is available in most healthfood shops and some supermarkets. As a rule you can replace traditional mince, in a bolognese sauce or lasagne, with one-fifth TVP without noticing the difference in the flavour. In spicy dishes like chillies, tacos or curries, you could probably use even more TVP without detracting from the flavour. As TVP has a much lower fat content than meat, this is a good way of reducing your fat intake and at the same time consuming a little soya. It is also a rich source of isoflavones, protein, calcium, iron and zinc, and contains few calories. In its dry state it has a long shelf life, but should be kept in a sealed container to keep moisture out.

Tofu

Tofu is the most widely known soya food amongst non-vegetarians, but not one that has gained broad popularity in the West, probably because most omnivores haven't much idea about how versatile tofu is and how it should be prepared. In Asian countries, tofu is almost associated with sacredness, as it is thought that it was first brought to China by Buddhist monks over 2,000 years ago and subsequently consumed by the upper classes. It is reported to have made its way to Japan by about AD 700. Today in China and other Asian countries, tofu is a fundamental part of the diet for both the rich and poor, young and old. It has an average consumption of 100 to 125 grams per day (3–4 oz), and a nickname of 'meat without bones'.

Tofu, also known as bean curd, is often compared to cheese as it is made from soya beans in the same way that cheese is made from dairy milk. It is made from dried soya beans that are soaked in water, then crushed and boiled. Nigari, a seawater compound like sea salt, or calcium salt, making the tofu an excellent source of calcium, is then added to the liquid squeezed from the soya bean, the soya milk, to make it curdle. The fresh warm curds from the liquid are poured into square moulds and left for several hours until they become firm. Subsequently they are separated from the whey and compressed into blocks. Tofu is best stored in cool water to keep it fresh, as it is a perishable food which needs to be kept at 45 degrees Fahrenheit or below. It is advisable to change the water daily to keep the tofu fresh. When fresh it should smell slightly sweet. Tofu that is slightly past its best can be freshened up by being boiled for ten minutes. Although tofu does not have a long shelf life in the refrigerator, it does keep well for up to five months in the freezer. After being frozen it often becomes darker in colour and takes on a spongier texture.

There are numerous types of tofu, suitable for different dishes, varying from firm tofu, softer versions which contain extra fluid and thus have a creamier consistency, usually known as silken tofu, and even freeze-dried products, which have a much more spongy texture. Tofu has a particularly bland flavour, and is probably so very versatile because it readily absorbs the flavour of food with which it is being cooked. You can make it taste like practically anything, and easily fool the most discerning palate. Firm tofu can be cubed or cut into strips for stews, stir-fries, kebabs, chillies and sauces. It can even be grilled or used as a replacement for scrambled egg! The silken tofu is best suited to creamy sauces, dips, pie fillings, whips, desserts, shakes, ice creams and cheesecakes, which are absolutely delicious. There is a variety of suggested recipes incorporating the different soya products, ranging from savoury meals to desserts and delicous creamy shakes. Turn to the recipe section starting on page 179.

Yuba

This soya product, which is a delicacy in China and Japan, is made from the skin that forms on the surface of soya milk when it is heated. It is carefully removed and then dried in sheets. Once dried it has a brittle consistency ideally suited to confectionery. It is also used to wrap vegetables and rice once it has been softened with water. Yuba is not currently widely available in the West, but you could always try making your own!

Yogurt

The food industry uses soya milk to make soya yogurt, by adding a bacterial culture in the same way that dairy yogurt is prepared. Although the taste of soya yogurts may have been lacking in years gone by, these days they are quite delicious. With some products like So Good, Naturally Good and Provamel's Yofu it is truly hard to tell them apart from dairy yogurts. It is worth trying out the brands that are available in your local healthfood shops and possibly even in your supermarkets.

YOUR DAILY DOSE OF LINSEEDS

Linseed oil

The recommended daily dosage of cold-pressed linseed oil is one tablespoon for every 45 kilos (100 lb) of body weight. It is probably best to begin with a smaller quantity and gradually build up to the full dose over a period of a few weeks. It can be used in salad dressings, drizzled on to vegetables including baked potatoes, on to fresh bread or taken with fruit juice. Always buy organic oil, ideally in a special darkened container that has been flushed with inert gas to exclude oxygen. Check the label, as it should be pressed at temperatures no higher than 33 degrees Centigrade. Once the bottle is opened it should be kept in the refrigerator for up to three weeks. Linseed oil should not be heated or used for cooking.

Linseeds

Fresh organic golden linseeds, which are much nicer than the brown seeds that are available, can be combined with breakfast cereal each day. Two tablespoons of seeds, either whole, or preferably ground (to release the oil), should be sprinkled over cereal, or used in muesli as an ingredient (see page 183). They can be ground either in a coffee grinder or a blender, or simply with a pestle and mortar, and then stored in a sealed container in the refrigerator to prevent rancidity. They can also be sprinkled over salads, including fruit salads, bakes, combined with yogurt or milk, and even included when baking fresh bread. It is important to consume plenty of liquid with linseeds, so if you are not combining them with milk, juice or yogurt have a drink afterwards.

The Cherokee Indians used to combine linseeds with curdled goat's cheese, cooked pumpkin and honey. Although this may sound like a strange combination, today's science tells us that this combination forms a special lipoprotein, a combination of oil and protein, which is acknowledged to have medicinal properties. Lipoproteins are known to help transport oxygen around the body, as well as being essential for the production of red blood cells and for fighting infection. By combining linseeds with either yogurt, preferably soya yogurt or soya milk, or tofu, or other sulphur-containing proteins like buckwheat, garlic or onion, you can increase your general health prospects as well as your intake of phytoestrogens!

There are many other plant-based foods that contain phytochemicals and, in particular, phytoestrogens. As science is yet young, we are unsure about how much isoflavone content many of them actually have. The following list of foods has been compiled as a result of wide reading over the last few years.

The benefits of legumes

In addition to soya products and linseeds, you will see from the chart on page 68 that chickpeas, lentils, mung beans and aduki beans are amongst the legumes that contain substantial levels of all four major isoflavones, including formononetin and biochanin, as well as daidzein and genistein. We can reap the benefit of their powerful isoflavone content by including them in our diet on a regular basis. They have been incorporated into the sample menus and recipes in Part Two, as an example of the different forms in which they can be enjoyed.

Foods rich in Isoflavones (mg/100 g)

Food	Isoflavones (mg/100 g)	Daidzein (mean)	Genistein (mean	Reference
So Good soy beverage	25	5	16	Sanitarium
Provomel soy drinks and desserts	12	N/A	N/A	Provamel
Soya beans (mature, cooked, boiled without salt)	54.66	26.95	27.71	USDA*
Soya beans, mature seeds, sprouted, raw	40.71	19.1	21.6	USDA*
Soya beans, flakes (defatted)	125.82	36.97	85.69	USDA*
Soybean paste	31.52	15.03	15.21	USDA*
Soya flour (defatted)	131.9	57.47	71.21	USDA*
Silken tofu (Vitasoy soft)	29.24	8.59	20.65	USDA*
Tofu (firm, prepared with calcium sulphate and nigari)	24.74	9.44	13.35	USDA*
Tofu (raw, ordinary, prepared with calcium sulphate)	23.61	9.02	13.6	USDA*
TVP (Textured Vegetable Protein)	22.9	7.9	11.8	Tham et al, 1998

Food	Isoflavones (mg/100 g)	Daidzein (mean)	Genistein (mean	Reference
Tempeh, cooked	53.0	19.25	31.55	USDA*
Tempeh burger	29.0	6.4	19.6	USDA*
Miso	42.55	16.13	24.56	USDA*
Miso soup mix, dry	60.39	24.93	35.46	USDA*
Soya protein isolate	97.43	33.59	59.62	USDA*
Soya cheese, unspecified	31.32	11.24	20.08	USDA*
Soya noodles, flat	8.5	0.9	3.7	USDA*
Soya & linseed bread (Vogel's)	37.9	N/A	N/A	Stevens & Co Australia
*Prevacan cereal bar (soya and flaxseed)	33.6 mg per bar	12.8 mg per bar	17.6 mg per bar	Phytogenics Limited
[*Inconclusive at time of going to press]				

* USDA-Iowa State University Database on the Isoflavone Content of Foods (1999). Website address: www.nal.usda.gov/fnic/foodcomp/Data/isoflav/isoflav.html
N/A = Figures not available

Foods rich in Lignans (mg/100 g)

Food	Lignans	Reference
Linseeds (flaxseeds)	371	Mazur 1998
Linseeds (flaxseeds)	59 mg per tablespoon	Mazur 1998
Pumpkins seeds	21.37	Adlercreutz & Mazur 1997
Bramble	3.74	Mazur 1998
Strawberry	1.58	Mazur 1998
Lingonberry	1.51	Mazur 1998
Cranberry	1.054	Mazur 1998
Otaheite gooseberry	3.05	Mazur 1998
Prevacan bar	3 mg per bar	Phytogenics Ltd
Chinese green tea	3.085	Mazur 1998
Prince of Wales black tea	2.725	Mazur 1998
Earl Grey black tea	1.787	Adlercreutz & Mazur 1997
Chinese black tea	1.14	Mazur 1998

Foods rich in Coumestans, Formononetin and Biochanin A (mg/100 g)

Food	Coumestrol	Formononetin	Biochanin A	Reference
Red clover		13220	8330	USDA*
Alfalfa sprouts	0	261	0	USDA*
Alfalfa sprouts mixed with clover sprouts	466	1771	2946	USDA*
Soya sprouts	38.6	0		USDA*
Clover sprouts	28.1	2.28	0.44	USDA*
Chinese peas, cooked	0	0	9.31	USDA*
Split peas, round	8.11	0	0	USDA*
Pinto beans, dry	3.61	Trace	0.56	USDA*
Garbanzo beans, dry	0	0.14	1.78	USDA*
Black-eyed beans, dry	0	0	1.73	USDA*
Pink beans, dry	0	1.05	0	USDA*
Mung beans, dry	0	0.61	0	USDA*
Split peas, yellow and green	0	0	0.86	USDA*

* USDA-Iowa State University Database on the Isoflavone Content of Foods (1999). Website address: www.nal.usda.gov/fnic/foodcomp/data/isoflav/isoflav.html

Many foods have been cited as having a phytoestrogen content, but at this time analyses of the actual isoflavone content has only been carried out on certain foods. After reviewing all the research, the advice we give at WNAS is to consume one good serving of soya per day, preferably tofu, tempeh, soya flour, soya protein isolate or soya beans, and one to two tablespoons of organic golden linseeds. In addition, ideally incorporate as many of the foods from the charts above as you can, on a regular basis. We have had tremendous success, over many years, in controlling hot flushes and helping to regenerate the lining of the vagina, by including phytoestrogen-rich foods into the diets of menopause patients. The sample menu plans outlined in Part Two of this book reflect our recommendations and I suggest you use them as a guideline until you have established your new regime. Now let's take a look at how phytoestrogens affect specific health problems.

A NEW BREED OF PHYTOESTROGEN-RICH SUPPLEMENTS

Both the pharmaceutical and the healthfood industries are aware of the scientific evidence regarding phytoestrogens helping to reduce symptoms of the menopause and protecting our bones from osteoporosis, as well as helping to control numerous other medical problems. They are also aware that Western women will not find it easy to change their eating habits quickly, to include the Japanese equivalent of phytoestrogen on a daily basis. With this in mind, they have set about solving the problem by producing supplements that provide isoflavones and lignans. The first wave of supplements are now on the market in Australia, the UK and the USA.

The rate at which new phytoestrogen- – or more properly isoflavone-rich – supplements are coming on to the market, makes it obvious that this is a commercial opportunity not to be missed. The result of this is a complicated marketplace, which more often than not doesn't deliver what it promises, although sometimes we may even get more for our money than we first imagined. Let me give you the lowdown of how to select a scientifically based isoflavone supplement that is likely to have a positive rather than a negative effect.

The majority of the first wave of supplements were soya-based pills. Now, the Japanese are not known for pill popping; rather they derive their 30–100 mg of phytoestrogens per day from their traditional diet. For soya-based supplements to genuinely have the ability to replace soya in the diet, they probably need to contain the correct ratio of genistein and daidzein. Also, they need to be derived from soya that can be guaranteed free of genetically modified ingredients. Many of the soya-based supplements are not standardised, they are not necessarily formulated with the correct ratios of phytoestrogens to mimic food supplied by Mother Nature, and they cannot realistically be guaranteed GMO free. Whilst not all soya-based supplements may fall into these categories, current research shows that, when selecting phytoestrogen-rich supplements, we chould err on the cautious side. According to Professor Kenneth Setchell, one of the most prolific researchers on the subject of phytoestrogens, from the Children's Hospital and Medical Centre, Cincinnati, we should stick to soya-based foods, rather than use supplements as a substitute. He has recently completed an analysis of 15 soya-based supplements and found that many of the supplements studied either did not contain what the label stated in terms of isoflavones, which would render them ineffective, or contained levels that would deliver higher doses of isoflavones than we would expect to find in a traditional Asian meal.

When looking for an isoflavone-rich supplement to include on the WNAS menopause programme, we chose a standardised and scientifically based product, which contains extracts from the root of the red clover plant. As the discovery of isoflavones is relatively recent, and still the subject of much ongoing research around the world, we decided not to rely on just one sort of isoflavone, but instead to recommend including a variety of isoflavone-rich plants into our regime. And, so far it seems to have paid off, as you will see from Chapter 9, Managing the Menopause Naturally, on page 78.

Novogen Red Clover

The first scientifically based supplement I became aware of was through an article in the *Sydney Morning Herald*. It is a product called Novogen Red Clover, which is made from the herb red clover, containing high concentrations of the isoflavones genistein, daidzein, formononetin and biochanin. Red clover is the richest known source of those four oestrogenic isoflavones, having up to ten times the levels of the next richest source, soya. Each 500 mg tablet of Novogen Red Clover is designed to deliver the same dose of isoflavones as a vegetarian diet based on legumes, approximately 40 mg of the four isoflavones. Two separate studies in Sydney, one at the Royal Hospital for Women and the other at the Royal North Hospital, have found that Novogen Red Clover reduces hot flushes and mood swings within eight weeks. Unlike drugs it does not seem to have side effects and offers women a herbal alternative at the time of the menopause. Our first study of the achievements of 100 menopausal patients who included this supplement in their regime, containing 40 mg of isoflavones per tablet, were very encouraging. We found that 75 per cent of the patients were totally symptom-free after following the WNAS programme for an average of four months. Further details of the menopause study can be found in Chapter 9 starting on page 92.

The choice of food or pills

Many women prefer to self-help with food rather than pills, but at least it seems they can choose which avenue to take. Those suffering with severe symptoms may choose to use a combination of pills and food initially, while their symptoms are at their worst. Although it is fine for all women and even children to consume phytoestrogen rich foods, it is not recommended that pregnant women, those breast feeding, or children take phytoestrogen supplements of any description. For details about the optimum daily dose of isoflavones see page 67.

As women now live, on average, until their mid-eighties, it is important to maximise the quality of health. Fortunately there are now many scientifically based self-help measures which, when implemented, will undoubtedly improve long-term well-being without any side-effects.

At the WNAS, we are very proud of our success rate in helping menopausal women. Within four months of following our programme

90 per cent of women report relief from the 'physical' and 'mental' symptoms, and 85 per cent are free from the oestrogen-withdrawal symptoms. In addition, the majority of women agree that once they have adjusted to the programme it is a most enjoyable way of life. So there really is no longer a need to suffer either the symptoms of the menopause, or the side-effects of HRT. Further details about the self-help plan for the menopause, with suggested menus and recipes, can be found in my book *Crusing Through the Menopause*.

At the WNAS, over the last 17 years, we have pioneered a scientifically based natural alternative to combat menopause symptoms. HRT is designed to help only the symptoms resulting from oestrogen withdrawal and does not address the physical and mental symptoms. Our programme, which is based on published medical papers, includes the use of phytoestrols, educates women about their bodies' needs and empowers them to help themselves to better health both in the short and the long term. This includes protecting themselves against heart disease and osteoporosis, as will be seen from the relevant chapters on these subjects.

8

THE NORMAL MENSTRUAL CYCLE

For women of child-bearing age, hormones can make or break their day, often accounting for why women may feel energetic, sexy and alert one day, yet irritable, aggressive and exhausted on other days of the monthly cycle. They have turned out to be far more powerful than we ever perceived. Some of the hormones currently written about in newspapers and magazines have a wide range of functions within the body and can very much influence the quality of our lives. These include adrenaline, which helps deal with stress, endorphins, the brain chemicals, which give us 'the feel good factor', and serotonin, the fashionable hormone, which helps to control mood and appetite. In fact, modern anti-depressants are designed to raise levels of serotonin in the brain, although serotonin levels can be raised naturally by consuming foods that contain high levels of the amino acid tryptophan, like bananas and whole grains. Our built-in hormone clock not only influences our brain, but other important functions like heart rate, blood pressure and body temperature.

Other hormones, including oestrogen and progesterone, although perhaps not so trendy, do pretty much overshadow all other hormones when it comes to the menstrual cycle and our fertility. Additionally, oestrogen is largely responsible for the youthful appearance of skin, hair and nails. The falling levels of oestrogen that we experience at the time of the menopause and beyond account for the accelerated ageing appearance of our skin, and the aches and pains that descend upon us at that time.

The menstrual cycle can be divided into two distinct halves. The follicular phase, which is the first half of the cycle, when the egg follicle is developing, and the luteal phase, the second half of the cycle, which occurs after ovulation. Oestrogen controls the first half of the cycle until the egg leaves the ovary, and progesterone is in control of the cycle from the day the egg is released until the menstrual period begins.

The normal age at which periods begin has been decreasing at a rate of three years per century. Currently, they usually commence between the tenth and sixteenth year in 95 per cent of girls. The menstrual cycle is simply a fertility cycle, which enables a woman to conceive a child. This cycle is repeated each month, and if fertilisation fails to occur a menstrual period results, which is the shedding of the lining of the womb in preparation for the next cycle. The length of a normal menstrual cycle can vary from approximately 22 days up to 34 days, with the first day of bleeding being counted as the first day of the cycle. It is the pituitary gland in the brain that controls the ovaries, by sending instructions to produce eggs each month and release them.

Hormones are produced by both the adrenal glands and the thyroid. The ovaries produce the sex hormones, the adrenal glands produce sex hormones and other hormones related to stress, and the thyroid gland produces its own hormones that control the body's rate of metabolism. These three glands are all controlled by the pituitary gland. The pituitary gland, which is like the conductor of the hormonal orchestra, stimulates the production of two important hormones, follicle stimulating hormone (FSH), and luteinising hormone (LH). Largely, these two hormones dictate the amount of the two very special sex hormones, oestrogen and progesterone, produced by an adult female.

THE NORMAL MENSTRUAL CYCLE

- **Between days 1 and 7** – during the menstrual cycle both oestrogen and progesterone levels are low, although oestrogen levels are beginning to rise.
- **Between days 7 and 14** – oestrogen levels continue to rise, peaking at the point of ovulation when the egg is released by the ovary, which usually occurs between the eleventh and fourteenth day of the cycle. Women are at their most fertile during this phase, and often look and feel at their best, as well as at their most sexy, with increased levels of libido.
- **Between days 14 and 21** – although oestrogen levels may remain stable during this time, levels of progesterone, the pregnancy hormone, rise rapidly in preparation for nurturing a fertilised egg.
- **Between days 21 and 28** – if conception fails to occur, both oestrogen and progesterone levels fall dramatically, resulting in a monthly bleed. Women who experience premenstrual syndrome (PMS) usually experience it during this phase. Details about how to overcome PMS can be found in my book *No More PMS!*

What can go wrong?

There are a number of events that can cause the hormones to become unbalanced. These include nutritional deficiencies, stress, disturbed gut function, poor liver function or even genetic predisposition. The result of a hormone imbalance can include:

• Premenstrual syndrome
• Heavy bleeding
• Irregular bleeding
• Mid-cycle spotting
• The growth of fibrous growth within the uterus, known as fibroids
• Endometriosis, when the lining of the womb grows outside around other organs
• Breast problems, including pain and the development of fibrous tissue
• Hyperprolactinaemia

EFFECTS OF DIET ON THE MENSTRUAL CYCLE

Since the 1930s, researchers have been looking at ways in which diet affects the monthly cycle. It emerges that there are numerous aspects of dietary intake that can have a dramatic influence on hormone levels, and as a result our general sense of well-being. When an unbalanced diet exists, or nutritional deficiencies are present, the whole system may become disturbed or more sensitive. If there is a severe reduction in calorie intake, for example, and the body weight falls to an unhealthy level as a result, the function of the pituitary gland will decrease and periods may cease altogether, or alternatively may continue, but without ovulation occurring. This is Mother Nature's way of protecting a woman from becoming pregnant by enforced contraception when her body is in an unhealthy state.

The hormones produced by all the hormone-producing glands do appear to be influenced by the type of diet we consume, our nutrient intake, and our level of exercise and stress.

« Frankie's Story »

Frankie Ferguson is a 36-year-old personnel manager who is also a single parent of one young child.

I had suffered with PMS for some time but my symptoms became particularly bad after the birth of my son. For the week or sometimes two before my period it felt like my brain was gone. I would be so aggressive with my son, less tolerant of mistakes he made than I would be normally and at work my customers and employees were treated with far less patience and tolerance as I felt so aggressive. I felt that I was wasting two weeks every month, particularly at work as my productivity and creativity was at an all-time low. I would want to sleep more and hide away. I read about the work of the WNAS in Me magazine and approached them for help. I was given a diet, supplement and exercise programme to follow, which I followed as closely as I could, plus I started going to exercise classes with my sister. Gradually things began to improve. My cycle went from being completely erratic to a regular 30-day cycle which was great in itself. The fatigue lifted and I began to feel calmer and more in control.

I began my programme six months ago and I can honestly say I feel so healthy now, so laid back I could almost fall over. I continue to include the plant foods into my diet which contain oestrogen, and I still take regular exercise. Life at home is normal again and I am managing far better at work. My colleagues have noticed that there has been a big change and in fact, I have just won the Employee of the Month Award out of 100 staff members. It is the first time our company has run this scheme so I was particularly pleased to be chosen. I received a cheque for £100 and a bottle of champagne but the best gift of all was that I found myself again.

Our nutrient intake

Specific levels of important nutrients are needed for brain chemical metabolism and normal hormone function. Vitamin B6, vitamin C, the minerals magnesium and zinc and essential fatty acids, have been shown to be subtly involved in the way in which the body responds to or processes the hormones that relate to the normal menstrual cycle. Our own research at the WNAS, in three separate studies, has confirmed that between 50 and 80 per cent of women with premenstrual syndrome have low levels of red cell magnesium. Low levels of B vitamins, particularly vitamin B6, have been associated with reduced clearance rates of oestrogen by the liver.

The role of fibre in the normal menstrual cycle

It has been observed that women consuming a vegetarian diet excrete more oestrogen through their bowel motions than meat eaters (omnivores). Other researchers found that vegetarians had significantly less oestrogen in their urine compared to meat eaters, who were consuming little in the way of plant fibre. It therefore seems that a low-fibre diet allows oestrogen to be reactivated in the gut, through the absence of friendly bacteria that are derived from plant fibre, rather than being excreted in the desired way through the bowel motions. Soya, linseeds (flaxseeds) and fruits, cereals, beans and vegetables are all rich sources of fibre.

Phytoestrogens

Because phytoestrogens are able to compete successfully for the receptor sites inside cells, they have the ability to normalise oestrogen levels within the body. Fascinatingly, they are able to raise a low oestrogen level and lower an elevated level into the normal range. Studies have shown that women consuming 45 mg of soya isoflavones per day lowered their levels of both luteinising hormone and follicle stimulating hormone, with a significantly increased follicular phase of their cycle. This delayed the progesterone peak, which is particularly useful if you have a short menstrual cycle. Another recent study found that the hormones oestradiol and progesterone decreased and once again the menstrual cycle was prolonged. Even within the space of four to eight weeks, women with previously short menstrual cycles were experiencing significantly longer cycles, with up to a three-day extension.

Organic linseeds (flaxseeds), rich in lignans, are also able to bring about changes in the menstrual cycle by prolonging the luteal phase and increasing the number of cycles in which ovulation occurs. A diet rich in unsaturated fatty acids from oily fish, herring, mackerel, pilchards, salmon and sardines, and organic linseeds, which are all rich sources of omega-3 fatty acids, helps to increase the uptake of hormones by the receptor sites on the surface of the cells.

Although research is young in this area, there is no evidence to show that phytoestrogens have a detrimental effect on fertility, in fact the reverse. Since we have been incorporating phytoestrogen-rich foods into our regime at the WNAS we have certainly noticed that women who were previously experiencing short cycles were happily reporting that the length of their cycle had regulated.

Phytoestrogens have also been shown to increase sex hormone binding globulin (SHBG), compared to the Western diet which is acknowledged to decrease it. Adequate SHBG levels are also an important aspect of the normal menstrual cycle, as they control how much oestrogen and testosterone is carried around the body.

THE EFFECT OF LIFESTYLE ON OUR HORMONES

Physical and emotional stresses have a powerful effect upon the menstrual cycle. Excessive exercise, if continued on a regular basis, may cause the pituitary to 'switch off' the ovaries. Thus periods cease and the levels of the sex hormone oestrogen may fall. This phenomenon is often experienced in competing athletes and ballet dancers, who as a result of their decreased levels of oestrogen are at much higher risk of experiencing fractures and premature thinning of the bones, osteoporosis. Emotional stress, such as the worry of becoming pregnant from having unprotected sexual intercourse, can itself lead to the delay or the missing of a period, which in turn increases the worry or the stress.

There is no doubt that eating a nutritious diet, rich in plant oestrogens, low in animal fat and refined produce, plus regular exercise will improve health and well-being generally. Research is now pointing very strongly to the fact that this way of life will also affect many aspects of hormone health, normalising our menstrual cycle, keeping premenstrual syndrome at bay, as well as the other unwanted symptoms and side-effects of hormone imbalance.

While a plant-rich diet seems to produce results, it is not necessary to convert to a vegetarian diet, but simply to include more soya, linseeds and other plant-based foods into your existing diet. The four-week recommended diet plan in Part Two explains what is required, and there are suggested menus for you to follow.

9

MANAGING THE MENOPAUSE NATURALLY

For at least three-quarters of all women in the Western world, the menopause brings with it rapid changes and unwanted symptoms, often disrupting life and causing utter misery. Frequent hot flushes during the day and sweats at night, result in exhaustion, disorientation and despondency. A dry vagina and reduced libido can wreck sex lives, and repeated insomnia can leave women wondering whether life, as they knew it, is over.

The menopause is a transition, which signals the end of a woman's monthly fertility cycle, and in order to have a smooth passage through it, our bodies need to be in really good shape.

WHAT IS THE MENOPAUSE?

The menopause itself is merely the day menstruation stops, which one can only usually be certain about with hindsight. Therefore many women experience the actual menopause without really knowing at the time. Most of the symptoms experienced occur during the peri-menopausal stage, which means 'around the time' of the menopause.

After the age of 40, the supply of eggs diminishes, and the level of the female hormone oestrogen begins to decline. The dwindling number of eggs then matures irregularly, so that as the menopause approaches, the length of the menstrual cycles start to vary and periods become irregular.

Periods cease when eggs run out. As oestrogen levels fall, the lining of the womb loses its main source of stimulation and periods stop altogether. The majority of women will have their last natural period somewhere between the ages of 45 and 55, with the average standing at just over 50. In rarer cases women start an early menopause in their late twenties or early thirties, and sometimes women continue having periods until they are in their late fifties.

KEY SYMPTOMS

From a survey conducted by the Women's Nutritional Advisory Service (WNAS), of 500 women who had recently gone through their menopause, it was discovered that there were three main groups of symptoms that occur at the time of the menopause. However, only one group is directly related to the falling oestrogen levels. The other two groups of symptoms, 'physical' and 'mental', are more related to dietary and lifestyle inadequacies.

Oestrogen-withdrawal symptoms:

These are predominantly:

- Hot flushes
- Night sweats
- Vaginal dryness
- Loss of libido
- Urinary symptoms
- Skin changes
- Difficulties with intercourse

Physical symptoms:

These consisted primarily of:

- Muscle aches and joint pains
- Irritable bowel syndrome
- Constipation
- Fatigue and tiredness
- Migraines and headaches

Mental Symptoms:

These include:

- Anxiety
- Panic attacks
- Palpitations
- Irritability
- Aggressive feelings
- Mood swings
- Depression and confusion
- Insomnia
- Poor memory
- Loss of concentration

All of the symptoms listed are commonly experienced. What is not widely appreciated, however, is that HRT is only aiming at the oestrogen-withdrawal group, and not necessarily the 'physical' and 'mental' groups of symptoms.

Nutrients lacking

It was discovered from research conducted by the WNAS on several groups of younger women suffering with premenstrual syndrome, that minerals like magnesium and iron and the B vitamins are often in short supply, which affects the efficiency of brain chemistry and hormone function. The menopause is a major transition, which places extra demands on brain chemistry. If the body is not working efficiently because of previous dietary inadequacies and lack of education, it is unlikely that you will experience a smooth passage.

What your doctor has on offer

The favoured treatment for menopausal women is Hormone Replacement Therapy (HRT). Oestrogen therapy was initially pioneered in the USA. Oestrogens alone were used for the first 20 years, but then it was discovered that women with an intact uterus had a greatly increased risk of cancer of the lining of the uterus, so progesterone was added to make it safer.

HRT – THE PROS AND CONS

Some women swear by HRT, but these are greatly outnumbered by the women who cannot tolerate it. Research shows that up to two-thirds of women who try HRT come off it within the first year, due to either side-effects or dissatisfaction. Because doctors are not widely educated about alternative treatments to HRT for women experiencing symptoms of the menopause, women are often left to fend for themselves.

A survey of 1,000 GPs also conducted by the WNAS shows that almost half the doctors experienced problems when prescribing HRT, and 43 per cent claimed that they experienced problems when treating menopausal women.

HRT RISK FACTORS

Large trials are underway to examine the actual risks attached to taking HRT. There are undoubtedly still recognised risks, and until these long studies are completed, which is likely to take another 20 years, the jury is still out. The following are the most serious of the risks.

Serious risk

- Increased possibility of breast cancer – in the region of 35 per cent after ten years on HRT

Don't take HRT if you have:

- A personal or close family history of cancer of the womb or breast
- Vaginal bleeding of uncertain cause

- Endometriosis (where the womb lining grows and subsequently bleeds outside the womb)
- A personal or strong family history of thrombosis (blood clots) especially if you are a smoker
- Severe cardiac, liver or kidney disease

HRT may also aggravate:

- Migraines
- Multiple sclerosis
- Epilepsy
- Diabetes
- High blood pressure (occasionally)
- Gall stones

The WNAS survey of doctors also showed a great inconsistency in prescribing alternatives to HRT, with some 36 different treatment approaches nominated; hardly surprising considering that 82 per cent of the GPs in the survey felt they had inadequate training on the nutritional approach to health, and a further eight per cent failed to answer the question.

HRT side-effects

(Compiled from data supplied by the manufacturers of HRT preparations and from the UK doctors' guide to drug prescribing.)

Less serious

- Gastro-intestinal upset
- Nausea and vomiting
- Weight gain
- Breast tenderness and enlargement
- Premenstrual syndrome symptoms such as mood changes
- Breakthrough bleeding
- Headaches or migraine
- Dizziness
- Leg cramps

Minor problems

- Increase in size of uterine fibroids
- Intolerance of contact lenses
- Certain skin reactions
- Loss of scalp hair
- Increase in body or facial hair

The risks of breast cancer defined

Another round of evidence published recently in *The Lancet* (Vol. 350, No. 9084, Saturday 11th October 1997), on the increased incidence of breast cancer with long-term usage of HRT must further the fear and confusion amongst women of menopausal age. As the pro-HRT lobby will continue to justify the figures, it is important to interpret the facts, cutting through the confusion.

The most recent publication was a meta-analysis of some 51 studies in 21 countries, which concluded that after 11 years' usage of HRT there is a 35 per cent chance of developing breast cancer. One of the main concerns is that the oestrogen in HRT increases the density of the breast tissue, thus making it much more difficult to detect abnormalities on a mammogram. This evidence is not exactly new, as both the British and American Cohort studies, which have been running for approximately 15 years, have also been showing worrying trends of increased breast cancer associated with long-term use of HRT. However, the new publication does bring it to the forefront of our minds.

The dilemma for women who are weighing up the pros and cons of taking HRT is their increased risk of heart disease, post menopause, without the protection of oestrogen. This is a real issue as current statistics show that some 30 per cent of women will develop heart disease, which until women reach the menopause is largely a male condition (Prof. Valerie Beral *et al.*, 'Breast cancer and HRT: collaborative reanalysis of data from 51 epidemiological studies of 52,705 women with breast cancer and 108,411 women without breast cancer'. *The Lancet* Vol. 350, No. 9084, Saturday 11th October 1997). The incidence of heart disease post-menopause, is far greater than the incidence of breast cancer on HRT, but for women breast cancer seems to be a more sensitive issue.

Despite the on-going pro-HRT campaigns by the Amarant Trust and others, only a small percentage, in the region of 11 per cent of menopausal women, are using HRT. Some doctors are more than eager to prescribe HRT to every patient over 40, which is understandable in a way as blood levels of oestrogen drop by about 60 per cent at the time of the menopause. However, there are other doctors, 23 per cent in a WNAS survey of 1,000 GPs, who are reluctant to prescribe it at all. Equally, according to the WNAS survey there is confusion amongst GPs as 53 per cent admit that they have difficulties treating menopausal women and 47 per cent are unsure about alternative methods of treatment. This is understandable as most of GPs' postgraduate training on the subject comes from the pharmaceutical industry, which is obviously a beneficiary of HRT sales.

The reason why women are reluctant to try HRT may be partly because of their previous hormonal experiences. Many of them may have developed side-effects such as weight gain, migraine and depression due to taking the high-dose oral contraceptive pill in their younger days. Some will later have been prescribed hormonal products for PMS, which quite often have side-effects. By the time they reach the menopause vast numbers of women are far from being 'hormonal virgins', which may explain why, despite their unwanted symptoms, they do not find the concept of taking HRT in the long term appealing.

Who really needs HRT?

The average age for menopause in the UK is approximately 51 years, but there are women who experience an early menopause most often because they are excessively thin, or smokers or have had a radical hysterectomy. Those who do experience an early menopause in their thirties or early forties are undoubtedly at greater risk of becoming victims of osteoporosis or heart disease.

As science stands at the moment there is a greater case for younger women, who experience a premature menopause, taking HRT than women who enter menopause in their late forties or early fifties who are of normal weight for their height and perhaps have no history of osteoporosis in the family.

WHAT YOU CAN DO

There is a great deal you can do to ensure a smooth passage through the menopause, whilst protecting your heart against disease and your bones against osteoporosis, without taking HRT. The following recommendations are used by the WNAS as part of our successful programme, and are all based on published scientific papers. Some examples follow of the power of the more natural approach to the menopause.

Phytoestrogens and the menopause

In 1990 a study published in the *British Medical Journal*, conducted by a group of Australian workers, showed that a group of women going through the menopause, regularly consuming foods and drinks that contained naturally occurring oestrogens, including soya products, organic linseed and a herb called red clover, were able to bring about the same positive changes in the lining of the vagina as women taking HRT. In 1992 a validation of how effective phytoestrogens are at the time of the menopause was published in *The Lancet*. The study concluded that Japanese women do not seem to experience hot flushes and other menopausal symptoms because the Japanese diet contains foods rich in plant oestrogens. These two studies spurred me on to include phytoestrogens in the WNAS menopause programme, and I have to say it has been a very successful action.

Much more exciting research has since been conducted on the effects of phytoestrogens to the point where it has been discovered that they have certain similarities to the 'designer hormones' the Selective Oestrogen Receptor Modulators, SERMS. These hormones are being developed to have a beneficial effect on the cardiovascular system and the skeleton, without having cancer-promoting effects on the breasts or the lining of the womb. However, unlike phytoestrogens, which help to relieve hot flushes, the down side with the SERMS is that they seem to cause hot flushes! There have been many positive studies on phytoestrogens and their role in controlling the oestrogen withdrawal symptoms of menopause.

For example, researchers at the University of South Manchester in England fed menopausal women a 60 gram soya protein drink daily for two months, which reduced hot flushes by half, and the remaining flushes were 30 per cent less severe. Another soya protein experiment was set up by Professor Burke, of the department of public health science at the Bowman Gray School of Medicine, Winston-Salem, North Carolina. He fed 43 American women, aged between 45 and 55, 20 grams of soya protein, sprinkled over their morning cereal, for six weeks. The women found that symptoms were significantly reduced, although they did not entirely disappear. As a result there is a larger ongoing study, whose subjects are being given much higher doses of soya.

In 1998 Dr Albertuzzi confirmed the value of soya protein in helping to control hot flushes. His study of 104 post-menopausal women, who took either 72 mg of isoflavones or a placebo each day for 12 weeks, showed that soya was significant in reducing the number of hot flushes experienced. Women taking soya found that their hot flushes decreased by 26 per cent after 3 weeks, 33 per cent by week 4, and 45 per cent by week 12, compared with a 30 per cent reduction in the hot flushes of women in the placebo group.

A few years ago, an Australian study of menopausal women consuming bread rich in both soya and linseeds, showed a 40 per cent reduction in hot flushes and a small increase in bone mass. This preliminary research indicates that these phytoestrogens may well be as powerful as HRT, not only in their effect on vaginal tissue, but also in protecting against both osteoporosis and heart disease. The soya and linseed loaf is now available in the UK in the form of the Burgen Loaf and Vogel's Soy & Linseed Loaf; in Australia it is available as the Burgen Soya-Lin Loaf; and in New Zealand as Country Fare Soya and Linseed Bread. The availability of this new bread makes it easier for many women in the Western world to include phytoestrogens in their diet on a regular basis, without having to change their eating habits. Four slices of these new loaves per day are designed to deliver a typical

Oriental or Asian daily serving of phytoestrogens to Western women. Other foods rich in plant oestrogens are now finding their way on to the market, including Wallaby bars, which are made by Energy Products. These are delicious snack bars, which contain soya beans and linseeds and are fortified with calcium. Prevacan bars, containing 33.6 mg of isoflavones per bar, are also new to the marketplace, and are a handy way of getting an instant 'phyto-fix'. Naturally, as the research in this area is so positive, we will find many other products on our shelves in the very near future. We need to be discerning however. Many foods may well contain phytoestrogen-rich ingredients in principle, but it is very difficult to standardise natural products. This became apparent to me after reading the results of a survey conducted by Novogen in Australia. The company analysed a long list of common phytoestrogen-rich foods including soya products, chickpeas and lentils, and found a terrific variation in phytoestrogen content. Amazingly, some of the tested foods contained very few phytoestrogens indeed. The phytoestrogen content of food may vary considerably depending on the crop, the time of year it was grown, the climate, and a number of other environmental factors. Foods that have been put through scientific analysis will state the phytoestrogen content on the label, so once again it is down to label reading, or alternatively you could bake some of the bread, fruit loaves, cakes or biscuits that are detailed in the recipe section, beginning on page 235.

It seems that Mother Nature has provided foods that allow us to top up our oestrogen levels, at the time of the menopause and beyond, quite naturally, without having to resort to Hormone Replacement Therapy. The only problem I have encountered is that women are generally unaware of which foods contain phytoestrogens; as a result our intakes in Western countries are negligible, compared to Asian women who consume between 50 and 100 grams of phytoestrogen or phytoestrogen-containing food per day.

Research so far does tell us about many of the foods that contain plant oestrogens and other important phytochemicals. Although we are beginning to know about the precise quantities of isoflavones and lignans in some foods, we have yet to determine the precise values of other foods. You will find the most up-to-date list of 'Phyto Foods' on page 55, and details about their values on the following pages. There are suggested recipes and menus for you to follow, which as you will see, suggest one serving of soya per day. Regular amounts of organic golden linseeds and many of the other phytoestrogens are woven through each day. Published research as well as our own findings point to the fact that a daily intake is necessary, preferably in split doses – in other words little and often – as these compounds leave the body fairly rapidly. It is thought that isoflavones reach a peak in our blood within approximately six to eight hours. We have certainly found that by consuming a phytoestrogen-rich breakfast, perhaps the phyto muesli outlined on page 165, together with So Good soya milk, and having a couple of additional 'phyto fixes', perhaps in the afternoon and evening, we can substantially increase the rate at which we can control menopausal hot flushes.

Whilst it seemed to be the general consensus of opinion of researchers presenting new data at the 3rd International Symposium on The Role of Soy in Preventing and Treating Chronic Disease (Washington D.C., 1999), that soya in our diet is only likely to decrease hot flushes by 30 per cent, our experience is that when combined with other aspects of the WNAS menopause programme, it is a valuable part of a highly effective, natural alternative to taking HRT, which aids the control of hot flushes in a relatively short time period.

As outlined in the phytoestrogen-rich foods section, unless you have the desire to change your diet radically, or are already a vegetarian, it is not necessary to make dramatic changes.

Whilst there are plenty of recipes for phytoestrogen-rich meals to be tried, you can just as easily get your daily phytoestrogen intake by combining So Good soya milk with fruit in the blender to make delicious fruit shakes, or blend silken tofu with fruit to make fruit whips. Additionally, there are savoury dips you can make that can be devoured with fresh vegetable *crudités* and corn chips, or you can sample a slice of our phyto fruit loaf for tea.

If you are aiming to overcome severe and debilitating symptoms at the time of the menopause, it is likely, in our experience, that you will need to consume at least 100 mg of isoflavones per day initially, combined with the other important aspects of the WNAS programme. This will enable you to emulate the Japanese in their consumption of daily phytoestrogens, but in a Western way.

" Nicola's Story "

Nicola is a 46-year-old mother of two and part-time conference organiser. She read about the WNAS in a national newspaper and contacted us as she was looking for an alternative to HRT because of the horrendous side-effects she had had from it.

At the age of 44, a blood test showed early menopause. I tried HRT but within days was experiencing panic attacks, depression, feeling totally out of control and suicidal. Within one week I had stopped the HRT and it took me several months to regain my composure. Apart from this, I was suffering from hot and cold flushes, night sweats, headaches, abdominal bloating, constipation, general aches and pains and continued depression.

At my initial clinic consultation with Maryon Stewart I was given recommendations with regard to my diet and supplements to take. I began the nutritional diet by avoiding wheat and bran, changing ordinary tea to Rooibosch tea and adding things like oily fish and phytoestrogen-rich foods and herbs. I was advised to take various supplements to boost my vitamin and mineral levels and help reduce my symptoms.

One month later I saw Maryon again at her clinic and was able to say that I generally had more energy and was more positive. My symptoms were reducing and I was satisfied with the nutritional diet. I travelled frequently with my job, staying in hotels but managed quite well to stick to the recommendations.

Four months down the line and I am getting on very well. I feel better mentally, more in control and much more positive. I am relaxing more now and will look into having some massage. My fatigue and irritability have gone. I am sleeping much better, my flushes are very infrequent and constipation is a thing of the past. A bonus throughout the programme at the WNAS is that my weight has dropped to a comfortable level for me at 55 kilos. I am very pleased with myself and people have noticed a more rational person in their midst.

USEFUL SCIENTIFIC FACTS

- Practising relaxation techniques for 15 to 20 minutes each day can reduce your hot flushes by as much as 60 per cent.
- Taking a magnesium-rich multi-vitamin and mineral supplement will help to put back into the body that which time and nature have removed.
- Taking supplements of calcium, essential fatty acids and marine fish oils can reduce the amount of calcium lost through the urine, increase the amount absorbed through the gut wall, and improve the calcium balance in the bones.
- Taking regular low-impact aerobic exercise like brisk walking, skipping, racquet sports or working out, is good protection against both heart disease and osteoporosis.
- A recent 12-week study conducted by a German doctor on 111 females with menopausal symptoms using the herbal treatment, Hypericum-Kira, showed that 60 per cent of the women regained

their libido, over 60 per cent also reported overcoming headaches, lack of concentration and palpitations, and a total of 80 per cent felt that their symptoms had improved or gone completely by the end of the study.

- Supplements of natural vitamin E, panax ginseng and dong quai have all been shown to help with the reduction of oestrogen withdrawal symptoms.

DIETARY RECOMMENDATIONS

Consume regular amounts of foods that contain plant oestrogens, phytoesterols, which Mother Nature in her wisdom has provided us with so that we can top up our oestrogen levels naturally on a regular basis (see page 55 for listing). It is well established, for example, that Japanese women, who already eat a diet particularly rich in phytoestrogens, have far fewer problems at the time of the menopause, and as mentioned previously until recently did not even have a term in their language for 'hot flush'.

1. **Reduce your intake of sugar and junk foods.** This includes sugar added to tea and coffee, and sugar in sweets, cakes, biscuits, chocolate, jam, puddings, marmalades, soft drinks containing phosphates, ice cream and honey. Consumption of these may impede the uptake of essential nutrients and may cause water retention.
2. **Reduce your intake of salt, both added to cooking and at the table.** Also avoid salted foods like kippers and bacon. Salt causes fluid retention and induces calcium loss from the body in the urine. Use potassium-rich salt substitutes and other flavourings such as garlic, onion, kelp powder, fresh herbs, sesame powder or other mild spices.
3. **Over-spicy food, hot drinks and alcohol can aggravate flushes.** Let hot drinks cool down and keep alcohol to a minimum whilst going through the menopause. Alcohol tends to impede the absorption of most nutrients which are important to conserve at this time.
4. **Eat vegetables and salads daily.** Three portions of vegetables and a salad should be eaten every day as they contain plenty of nutrients. Where possible use organic produce, or grow your own.
5. **Eat plenty of fresh fruit.** Eat at least two servings each day as fruits are good sources of nutrients.
6. **Limit your consumption of red meat to one or two portions each week.** Substitute meat with fish, poultry, peas, beans and nuts,

as meat eaters have a lower bone density than their vegetarian counterparts.

7. **Dairy products, such as milk and cheese, are good sources of calcium.** Use low-fat versions if you need to watch your weight. Aim to drink 600 ml (1 pint) of milk per day, or other foods rich in calcium, like unsalted nuts, bony fish, green vegetables, cheese, cereals and soya products.

8. **Keep consumption of animal fat to between 20 and 30 per cent of your total calorie intake.** For most this means reducing fat intake by at least one-quarter. Instead, use cold-pressed oils such as linseed, safflower, sunflower, olive, sesame, rapeseed etc., and use soft polyunsaturated spreads instead of hard margarines or lard.

9. **Drink plenty of liquids.** Preferably drink the equivalent of six glasses of water daily. Use decaffeinated drinks, or better still herbal alternatives.

10. **If you smoke, try to cut down gradually, or better still stop completely.** Smoking can aggravate symptoms, especially hot flushes and night sweats, and smokers tend to have an earlier menopause. Stopping smoking at the time of the menopause can reduce the risk of hip fracture, by as much as 40 per cent.

12. **Keep a supply of nutritious snacks to eat in between meals if you get peckish.** Unsalted nuts, raisins and fresh or dried fruit are fine.

《 Janice's Story 》

Janice is a 49-year-old beauty therapist and aromatherapist from Nottingham.

I suffered with significant menopausal symptoms for two years and had tried numerous HRT treatments, but because of the side-effects, stopped after ten months. I was suffering from hot and cold flushes, night sweats, a bloated abdomen, and had gained one stone in weight whilst I'd been on HRT. A great problem also was my lack of libido, which didn't help my relationship.

I read the book Cruising Through the Menopause, *and contacted the WNAS, as I preferred to try the natural approach. I had been following instructions from the book but needed advice about how to proceed and which supplements to take. During my first consultation I was given details of food products to avoid on a temporary basis and others to include such as foods and herbs containing naturally occurring oestrogens. Plus, I was advised to try to increase my exercise and to continue with my yoga, perhaps considering some massage. The supplements recommended were varied and each had a role to play on the path to my recovery. I was more than willing to follow the recommendations.*

My next consultation was approximately two months later. I had been under a great deal of stress, which made my progress slower, but my tummy was less bloated, and I did feel as though I was on a more even keel. I was relaxing more and exercising as well. Maryon suggested taking a hypericum (St. John's Wort) remedy, Kira, to help improve my libido, which I readily agreed to.

By my third consultation I was feeling brilliant and my symptoms were only mild. Stress was always present in my life but I was intrigued, as my symptoms didn't get worse. It wasn't until I was feeling so much better that I realised how badly I had felt before. Now I wanted to tackle some of the extra weight I had gained, and Maryon made other recommendations in this direction.

My confidence is back and I am in control. I keep being told how well I look having lost half a stone, which makes me feel even better. The libido is back and my relationship is better than it has been for a long time. I can't speak too highly of the WNAS.

OTHER USEFUL SELF-HELP TIPS

- Aim to exercise for at least half an hour five times per week – you need to do weight-bearing exercise that is also aerobic. The benefits are a healthy heart, strong bones and a feeling of well-being.
- Try to spend 15 to 20 minutes relaxing each day to keep the stress levels down and the flushes at bay. Research shows that these simple measures will reduce hot flushes by as much as 60 per cent.
- Wear several layers of thin, comfortable clothing during the day so that you can peel them off should the need arise.
- Use lightweight layers of bedclothes so that you can adjust them according to temperature. Wear cotton nightdresses instead of man-made fibres.
- Carry some cool wipes in your handbag until the flushes have abated.
- Take extra care of your hair, skin and nails; use rich hair conditioner, good moisturising lotions for your skin and nail strengtheners.
- Do toning pelvic-floor exercises once or twice a day by repeatedly holding in the vaginal muscles to the count of ten and releasing slowly.

THE VALUE OF SUPPLEMENTS

As only a relatively small percentage of menopausal women continue to take Hormone Replacement Therapy in the long term, the 'menopause market' is probably perceived as a gold mine by the manufacturers of non-drug products. In the USA there are an estimated 30 million menopausal women not taking HRT, only 4 per cent take it in Italy, whilst in the UK it is reckoned to be 15–20 per cent of all menopausal women (source: Amarant Trust, UK). Australian surveys show that approximately 30–40 per cent of menopausal women currently use HRT. You don't have to be a mathematician to work out that this means that there are millions of women world-wide looking for a solution to their menopause symptoms, usually independently of their doctors.

As discussed on page 69 the last few years has seen an abundance of mainly soya-based supplements coming to the marketplace. Sadly, the vast majority of these are not scientifically based, and according to research, are not necessarily likely to protect us in the same way as soya-based foods. In fact, eminent professors including Professor Kenneth Setchell and Professor Herman Adlercreutz, who are probably considered within research circles to be the fathers of phytoestrogens, are actively dissuading the use of soya-based supplements, until further research has been undertaken.

The Japanese traditionally consume soya products within their diet, in relatively small quantities, meaning that their isoflavone intake from soya is little and often. One of the dangers with soya-based supplements is that they are designed to give a large dose of isoflavones, in one dose. Studies have shown that these do not have the same effect as soya-based foods on symptoms of the menopause and preventing heart disease, for example.

But despite these findings there is a real need for an isoflavone-rich supplement, because realistically, the majority of Western women are not likely to adopt a similar diet to the Japanese. Whilst on the WNAS menopause programme we have successfully managed to disguise soya milk, soya flour and tofu within our recipes, which you will find in the menu and recipe section beginning on page 165. We aim to encourage women to consume many of the milligrams of phytoestrogens they require daily in the form of food. However, initially, when symptoms are severe and debilitating, we find great value in combining this with the use of a supplement. The supplement we use delivers 40 mg of the four main isoflavones per tablet, in the form of red clover, another isoflavone-rich substance, rather than soya. You will see from page 70 that the supplement of our choice is a scientifically-validated red clover preparation produced by the Sydney-based company, Novogen.

A recent US study has validated the effectiveness and safety of Novogen Red Clover (Promensil). The study, conducted by Tufts University School of Medicine and New York University School of Medicine, showed that menopausal women who took a single tablet of

Red Clover daily experienced a reduction in the intensity and number of hot flushes. Hot flushes were reduced by 56 per cent (from 8.1 per day to 3.6 per day) after 8 weeks. Intensity of hot flushes also decreased by 56 per cent, and night sweats decreased in intensity by 52 per cent. Hot flushes and night sweats are the two most common symptoms in menopausal women. The other good news was that Red Clover did not cause thickening of the endometrial lining, which is a complication commonly associated with HRT. The women in the study also reported no side effects or weight gain from taking the Red Clover.

We have now been using Novogen Red Clover as part of the WNAS menopause programme for the last two years. Within the first few months of experimenting with the product, which we did by giving samples to our patients to try, we discovered that the hot flushes and the night sweats were being controlled much more quickly. Whereas it used to take us at least three or four months to control hot flushes prior to using the Red Clover supplement, once we included the supplement into the programme we noticed that we were able to control the hot flushes much more quickly. Patients began returning for their follow-up appointment, just one month after their initial consultation, delighted that both their flushes and night sweats were far milder. This was excellent news to the WNAS team, as well as to the patients themselves, who were keen to be restored to normality as soon as possible.

The women included in the study had been suffering from menopausal symptoms for an average of almost four years, and their average age was 51 years. Thirty-seven of the women had previously tried HRT to help control their symptoms, of whom half had experienced side effects.

Results of the WNAS Menopause Programme incorporating Novogen Red Clover

Severe symptoms	Degree of improvement
Palpitations	95%
Insomnia	83%
Irritability	79%
Hot flushes	77%
Loss of confidence	72%
Dry vagina	70%
Night sweats	60%
Loss of libido	60%
Panic attacks	55%

Novogen Red Clover is available from many chemists and health food shops, and is also available from the WNAS mail order service; for details see page 265.

Redressing the balance

Through research over the years at the WNAS we have come to realise that the menopause is often the time when nutritional cracks appear. A combination of years of wear and tear, pregnancy and breastfeeding, challenge our nutrient stores, and the lack of knowledge about how to replace what time and nature have taken, leaves many women in a depleted state at the time of this important transition. Replacing the important nutrients including magnesium, zinc, B vitamins and essential fatty acids is vital for brain chemical metabolism as well as normal hormone function. In order to redress the balance, for more than 14 years we have been successfully using a magnesium-rich multi-vitamin and mineral supplement, called Gynovite, as part of the WNAS menopause programme. This supplement was formulated by a professor of obstetrics and gynaecology, and designed for women at the time of the menopause and beyond. It has been shown to positively influence brain chemistry and hormone function, and to help to improve our bone mass. Natural vitamin E has also been shown to be moderately helpful in helping to control the hot flushes.

Other herbs used to relieve symptoms of the menopause

- **Black Cohosh**, also known as *Cimicifuga racemosa*, is a native plant of North America that contains phytoestrogens. It was used by North American Indians to treat female disorders, including menopausal symptoms.
- **Dong Quai**, also known as *Angelica polymorpha*, also contains phyto-estrogens, and is considered in Chinese medicine as a harmonising tonic. It has traditionally been used to treat female complaints such as heavy bleeding and premenstrual syndrome, and now has a place in the treatment of menopause symptoms.
- **Liquorice root**, also known as *Glycyrrhiza glabra*, and **sarsaparilla root** also contain phytoestrogens. They are sometimes used in conjunction with other herbs in a mixture that can be brewed into a herbal tea. Liquorice can cause sodium retention and a risk of high blood pressure in some people.
- **Panax Ginseng** has been shown to be moderately helpful in controlling hot flushes, in our experience especially when used in conjunction with natural vitamin E. In fact, before we began using Novogen Red Clover, this was the combination of our choice. Ginseng is on the list of phytoesterols, the oestrogen-like substances. It comes in supplement form from healthfood shops, and can also be used in the form of ginseng tea.

- **Sage,** also known as *Salvia officinalis*, contains oestrogenic substances which can be helpful for the relief of hot flushes and night sweats.
- **St John's Wort** (*Hypericum*) has been used in the treatment of depression for many years, and is thought to be more effective in the treatment of moderate depression, and have fewer side-effects, than conventional anti-depressants. A 12-week German study of 111 women experiencing libido problems at the time of the menopause showed that 60 per cent of the women significantly regained their libido.

Further details about the WNAS menopause programme can be obtained from my book *Cruising Through the Menopause*.

10

PHYTOESTROGENS AND CANCER PREVENTION

Cancer is one of the commonest diseases of our time, and probably the most feared illness. Rightly so, for according to a World Health Organisation study on populations of some 50 countries, the incidence of cancer is much higher in industrialised Western societies than in Asian populations. For example, depending on which Western country you live in, your chances of dying from breast or prostate cancer are between ten to 20 times greater than people who have a typically Asian diet and live in countries like Japan, China or Thailand. At present, at least 20 per cent of the UK population will die of cancer, and it is thought that one in three in the UK will be affected by cancer at some stage in their lives. More than one in four people will have cancer during their lifetime and, after heart disease, cancer is the most common cause of death in Western countries, and the numbers are on the increase because of the ever expanding population. The peak incidence of adult cancer is after the age of 45. Sadly, we have reached the point where most of us have either a family member or friend who has become a cancer victim.

However, research now shows that cancer is not an inevitable disease, but one that seems to be more related to diet and environmental factors than to genetic disposition. To support this theory, let's look at what happens to the incidence of breast cancer when women move from Asia to the Western world and adopt the local diet.

Ten times more women currently die of breast cancer in England and Wales than in Korea, and Japan loses one-quarter fewer women to breast cancer than the United States. Research shows that when Asian women migrate and adopt Western eating habits, their statistics for cancer mimic those of the Western world in a relatively short period of time. In fact, the rate at which the statistics change is directly related to the speed and extent to which the dietary changes are made.

HOW DOES CANCER DEVELOP?

A cancerous growth may originate with only one, or a few cancerous cells that begin multiplying many months, or even years, before the victim perceives there is a problem. Cancerous cells have two main characteristics. They grow rapidly and multiply faster than the cells of the tissues in the surrounding area. In addition, they are able to spread, not just to local sites, but to tissues in distant areas. For example, a breast cancer victim may develop secondary sites in the lymph nodes under her armpit, and from there the cancer may travel to the liver or the spine. It is the speed at which the cancer multiplies and its widespread nature that results in death.

Risk factors for cancer

For the majority of cancers, increasing age, especially over the age of 40, is the greatest risk factor. In addition to this there are a number of known causes of cancer.

- **Cigarette smoking** is a widely acknowledged factor associated with increased risk of cancer. In fact, up to 30 per cent of all cancers are estimated to be linked to smoking. While its association with lung cancer is well known, what is not widely appreciated is that it is also associated with an increased risk of many other types of cancer, including of the mouth, throat, oesophagus, pancreas and bladder.
- **Excess levels of oestrogen** in the body encourage some ordinary cells to become cancer cells. High oestrogen levels can result naturally, with the help of synthetic oestrogen from preparations like Hormone Replacement Therapy, or indeed following exposure to environmental oestrogens as discussed on page 23.
- **Exposure to sunlight or ultra violet light** in white, especially fair-skinned, individuals is associated with skin cancer. Melanoma, a form of skin cancer, has become the commonest cause of death amongst young people in Australia and South Africa, as well as being on the increase in the United Kingdom.
- **Significant amounts of natural radiation** are a powerful invisible force that can disrupt the structure of cells, precipitating cancerous growth.
- **Some industrial chemicals** are also associated with an increased cancer risk. These include rubber, asbestos, glues, varnishes, cadmium, nickel, industrial dyes and some rare metals.
- **Certain viral infections** have also been associated with changes in cell structure that may lead to cancer of the cervix, the stomach and

even HIV. A virus is also capable of suppressing the immune system, which in turn increases the risk of cancer. These forms of cancer account for approximately 15 per cent of all cancers and are usually preventable. Eradication of the Helicobacter pylori germ, associated with peptic ulcers, may lead to the reduction of stomach cancer, so too will reducing the intake of pickled foods. Research also shows that reducing the number of sexual partners a woman has, especially before the age of 20, having a circumcised partner and using condoms are all examples of how to reduce the risk of cervical cancer.

- **Poor diet** is a major causative factor. High intakes of fat, especially saturated fats, are associated with increased risks of breast cancer, as well as cancer of the colon, endometrium (lining of the womb), pancreas and prostate. Research conducted in many countries around the world, including Australia, Europe and the USA, quite clearly shows that a diet rich in fruit and vegetable fibre, combined with phytoestrogens and low in saturated animal fats, offers a great deal of protection against most forms of cancer. A healthy diet is certainly necessary for normal immune function. Several studies have shown that vegetarians have higher levels of immune system cells, which are capable of killing both tumour cells and viruses.

Conventional medicine has become better at detecting cancer in the early stages and consequently more cancer victims are surviving than in past years, but it is currently a long way from offering a cure for most cancers. The direct costs of cancer are astronomical. In the USA it is estimated that the annual costs exceed $100 billion per year, and only 2 per cent of that is spent on research. Other costs include $35 billion per year for diagnosis and treatment, $12 billion per year for loss of productivity as a result of the illness, and approximately $57 billion per year resulting from loss of economic activity because of premature death. In Australia, cancer is the second highest cause of death, claiming the lives of 24 per cent of women and 27 per cent of men, and in the UK cancer is the cause of one quarter of all deaths.

How cancerous cells get started

The cells in the body are constantly dividing and reproducing. The approximately 100 trillion cells in the average body are likely to reproduce 10,000 billion times in a lifetime, which means that in every minute of every day about 10 million of your cells divide. Healthy cells are incredibly intelligent. They know precisely when it is time to grow or divide and when to stop, and this wisdom is known as 'the cell cycle'.

These microscopic cells are also exceptionally astute as they are able to differentiate. They know how a kidney cell should act, for example, compared to a brain or a breast cell.

Not all cells have the potential to become cancerous, only those known as stem cells are candidates, and although stem cells usually divide correctly, sometimes things go wrong. Unlike normal cells, cancer cells lose their ability to differentiate, they return anonymous looking cells that instead of performing the particular function of the parent cell simply grow and disrupt the activity of healthy cells around them. The rapidly developing mass is known as a tumour, which may either be benign (non-cancerous) or malignant (cancerous). When tumours or masses become sufficiently large, the adjacent organs fail to function properly and, if untreated, eventually death results.

The genetic material at the centre or nucleus of the cell determines our characteristics and is known as deoxyribonucleic acid (DNA). Its job is to give cells instructions about the production of proteins; among these are enzymes without which we could not survive. When a cell divides it usually makes an exact copy of the DNA to pass on to the daughter cell. Normally this process progresses without problems, but somewhere between 1 in a million and 1 in 100 million times a mistake occurs and the result can be a cancer cell. A damaged cell may lie dormant for many years or months before it is triggered to multiply. There is now strong scientific evidence to suppose that oestrogen encourages these 'damaged' cells to start dividing. Many studies have shown that when oestrogen attaches itself to the receptor site within a cell, it can stimulate the cell to divide and grow abnormally. It speeds up the cell cycle and interferes with the cell's normal growth mechanism. This theory is not new, however, as in the 1880s doctors observed that women with breast cancer, who had their ovaries removed, subsequently had shrinking tumours.

Although it is thought that in some cases cancer may have a genetic element, for example breast cancer is more likely to affect daughters of victims and colon cancer can pass through families, the majority are not genetically fated to become cancer victims. Instead, the diet, lifestyle and environment will determine how our cells reproduce and whether or not they become cancerous.

THE ROLE OF DIET

It has long been established that those consuming a diet rich in animal fats and low in fibre are more likely to develop cancer than those consuming a wholesome diet, rich in anti-oxidant nutrients (A, C, E and selenium). However, until relatively recently the medical profession has had its attention firmly on drugs to kill off cancer cells and possibly to boost the immune system. Surprisingly, massive amounts of research looking at the role of phytoestrogens in the prevention of cancer have been conducted by highly respected scientists, in reputable research units around the world. In fact, there is a vast amount of research material, much of which until now has not been translated from 'medicalese' into ordinary language for the public.

Lignans and isoflavonoids

Research has confirmed that plant lignans and isoflavonoids are converted by bacteria in the intestines to hormone-like compounds, with weak oestrogenic and anti-oxidative activity. They have been shown to influence many key functions within the body including:

- Sex hormone metabolism
- Biological activity
- Enzyme function
- Production of protein
- Growth factor action
- Malignant cell proliferation
- Cell differentiation
- Angiogenesis – the development of new blood vessels

Very recent research is suggesting that the dramatic reduction in cancer, which has been observed following regular consumption of phytoestrogens, may not be directly attributable to the foods themselves, but possibly to the chemical reactions that they bring about within the body.

Animal studies

There are literally hundreds of studies using phytoestrogens on animals, aimed at reducing the incidence of cancer; two-thirds of which show a dramatic reduction in the occurrences of cancer, and also the tumour size in those who had established cancer. Over 200 of these studies have looked at genistein, the soya isoflavone, alone as it seems to be able to influence many of the fundamental aspects of the cancer process. For example, one of the common enzymes produced by the genes that cause cancer (the oncogenes) is known as protein tyrosine kinase. In 1987, it was discovered that the isoflavone, genistein, in the form of soya, was actually a naturally occurring tyrosine kinase inhibitor, which means that it is able to prevent the activation of the specific genes that cause cancer. This it seems is just one of the counter-productive enzymes involved in the cancer process that genistein is able to constrain. It is interesting to note that Oriental populations, who have low rates of breast and prostate cancer, consume between 20 and 80 mg of genistein per day, almost entirely derived from soya products. Conversely, daily intakes of soya products in Western countries like Australia, the UK and the USA are almost negligible, between 1 and 3 mg per day.

Another attribute of genistein is that it seems to be able to inhibit the growth of blood vessels on which tumours depend for their supply of nutrients and oxygen. So as well as being a useful tool in the prevention of cancer, genistein may also have a part to play in treatment and it has been suggested that it may become one of the first of a new class of anti-cancer drugs. We don't have to wait for this particular new science to evolve, since we can get our daily genistein fix in the form of foods containing soya products.

Population studies

In addition to the animal studies there have been over 30 population studies conducted around the world looking at a wide variety of cancers and the response to many types of soya foods. The overall consensus is that those consuming soya products on a regular basis, probably daily, are likely to at least halve their chances of getting cancer, compared to those who eat soya products only once or twice per week. The studies show that the soya foods used were able to inhibit the growth of many types of cancer, including breast, prostate, colon, rectum, skin, lung, stomach as well as leukaemia. The vast majority of the studies identified the protective effects of soya products and golden linseeds (flaxseeds) in particular, and it is reassuring to note that there was no evidence reported in any study to suppose that these phytoestrogens could increase the incidence of cancer of any type.

One Japanese study showed that a whole range of soya products, including soya milk, soya protein, miso and tofu, were also able to block the formation of nitrites, the chemical compounds that are carcinogenic.

Golden linseeds

Golden linseeds (flaxseeds) are the richest source of lignans, and a regular intake has also been associated with low levels of cancer of the breast, the ovaries, uterus, prostate and the colon. Following consumption, they are readily excreted in the urine, which indicates that they are metabolised by the body. Researchers have shown that much higher levels of lignans are excreted by vegetarians than meat eaters, and one study found that very low levels of lignans were excreted by older women with breast cancer. Animal studies show that primates that excrete high levels of lignans rarely experience breast cancer.

As well as containing anti-cancer properties, lignans have been found to contain antifungal, antibacterial and antiviral properties.

So it seems that research of recent years on phytoestrogens has provided the key to lower the risk of cancer, therefore making the cure a less urgent issue for many of us. However, as well as consuming a daily serving of soya and regular amounts of other foods that contain phytoestrogen, which are outlined in Part Two, Eating for Health, it is important to ensure that other aspects of your diet and lifestyle are in order. You will find the key rules to general health and well-being outlined in my book *The Zest for Life Plan*, and in addition I have prepared a checklist for you to consider, which you will find at the end of this chapter.

PHYTOESTROGENS AND HORMONE-RELATED CANCER

Breast cancer

Breast cancer has historically been the commonest fatal cancer in women between the ages of 40 and 55, but unlike other forms of cancer, in recent years it has almost reached epidemic proportions in Western countries. In the USA for example, whereas in 1950 there was a one in 20 chance of women becoming breast cancer victims, today it has become a one in eight chance. This increase makes it now the leading cause of death in women between the ages of 40 to 55 years of age, and approximately a quarter of the women diagnosed with breast cancer each year will die. In Australia in 1990, apart from skin cancer, breast cancer was the most commonly diagnosed cancer. The highest breast cancer rates in the world are in North America, Northern Europe, Australia and New Zealand.

There are a number of contributory factors that have been found to be associated with breast cancer:

- A high consumption of animal fat and low-fibre diets, as found in many Western countries. Although the additional animal fat in the diet increases the intake of oestrogen, it is unlikely that this factor alone could account for such a consistent increase in breast cancer statistics.
- The absence of pregnancy or pregnancies after the age of 35. The risk is reported to be less likely with increasing numbers of pregnancies and episodes of breast feeding.

101

- Obesity, particularly in women after the menopause, as oestrogen is stored in the fat cells. Obesity is also reaching epidemic proportions. In the UK it is estimated that one in four people are overweight, one-third of the white adult population in the USA and Canada are obese, and according to a 1993 report, the direct cost of obesity in Australia in 1989–90 was $672 million. What is even more frightening is that children of obese parents are 70 per cent more likely to be obese themselves.
- Early onset of menstruation, which in theory means more hormonal cycles. This means more oestrogen production, which increases the chances of cancer.
- A family history of cancer, especially in a close relative such as a mother or sister. Many researchers have been concentrating their efforts on a search for a 'breast cancer gene', but this is not likely to apply to more than five per cent of victims.
- Fibrocystic disease of the breast.
- Constipation, which may affect hormone metabolism and the excretion of oestrogen.
- The oral contraceptive pill and injectable contraceptives carry a small increase in risk after prolonged use.
- Hormone Replacement Therapy (HRT) appears to increase the chances of suffering breast cancer by approximately 35 per cent following long-term usage, over five or ten years.
- Lastly, and probably most importantly, exposure to xenoestrogens – the environmental oestrogens discussed in Chapter 3.

It is thought that early life exposure to phytoestrogens may be critical for breast cancer prevention. Specifically, it is thought that genistein exposure pre-pubertally may decrease the risk of tumours in later life. There has been concern that soya isoflavones cannot yet be clearly stated as protective for breast cancer.

Recent research presented by Cline *et al* (3rd International Symposium on the Role of Soy in Preventing and Treating Chronic Disease, Washington D.C., 1999) looking at the effects of dietary soya on the uterus and breasts of female macaque monkeys, concluded that soya phytoestrogens do not stimulate the breast or uterine tissue. These monkeys are an accepted model for human female reproductive studies. These post-menopausal monkeys were fed either 148 mg of soya phytoestrogens per day for three years, or given oestrogen (1.25 mg per day). Cell proliferation (the growth and spreading of cancerous cells) was induced in monkeys given oestrogen but not soya phytoestrogens.

PHYTOESTROGENS – SOME BETTER NEWS

As phytoestrogens successfully compete for the oestrogen receptor sites within the body, over and above normal oestrogen and xenoestrogen, and it seems raise levels of sex hormone binding globulin, they are able to block out the excess levels of oestrogen thought to precipitate breast cancer. Many published studies show encouraging results. One study in Singapore compared 200 women with breast cancer with 420 without. It emerged that those with the lowest risk of breast cancer consumed about 55 grams of foods containing soya per day, and concluded that those with the highest soya consumption had less than half the risk of breast cancer than those who rarely consumed soya products. In another study, 142,857 Japanese women were followed for 17 years, and it emerged that those regularly consuming soybean paste soup had a much lower risk of experiencing breast cancer.

Linseeds (flaxseeds) have also been shown to reduce the incidence of breast cancer. They are rich sources of lignans, which bear a structural similarity to oestrogen, and can bind to oestrogen receptor sites and inhibit the growth of oestrogen-stimulated breast cancer. A recent publication in *The Lancet*, which was conducted by Dr David Ingram and colleagues from Perth, Australia, also found a substantial reduction in breast cancer risk among women with a high intake of phytoestrogens, particularly isoflavones and lignans.

Current research shows that phytoestrogens are unlikely to be sufficient to inhibit the growth of mature, established breast cancer cells, but it seems they will regulate the proliferation of the cancer cells, thereby having a chemopreventive effect. Research is young, and much still remains to be learned about the influence of specific dietary constituents and cancer risk, but it is clear that our diet does have a significant impact in cancer prevention and control.

Phytochemicals – guardians of our health

Fruit and vegetable consumption has also been linked to the reduction of breast cancer. A study of 2,400 Greek women noted that women with the highest intake of vegetables, four to five servings daily, had a 46 per cent lower risk of breast cancer compared with women who had the lowest intake, fewer than two servings per day. Foods and herbs which have been shown to have anti-cancer activity include garlic, ginger, liquorice, cabbage, carrots, celery, cilantro, parsley, parsnips, onions, linseeds, citrus, turmeric, broccoli, Brussels sprouts, cauliflower, tomatoes, peppers, brown rice and whole wheat.

« Carla's Story »

Carla was a 32-year-old mother of three from Bradford, who had a history of breast cancer. She approached the WNAS for help, as she was not a candidate for HRT.

I lost both my mother and my grandmother at the age of 56 from breast cancer. My own breast cancer was diagnosed at the beginning of 1994 for which I underwent a mastectomy. Following my chemotherapy I was put on a drug called Tamoxifen designed to prevent new cancerous cells, but unfortunately one of the side-effects I experienced were hot flushes. In June 1995 I was advised to have a radical hysterectomy, which involved removing my ovaries, to lower my chances of contracting other female cancers.

I was relieved to have lowered my risk of cancer, but after the operation felt very tired, with little vitality, and noticed that my hot flushes had become severe and debilitating. I knew that I was not able to take HRT because of the cancer, and therefore set about finding an alternative. I found the first edition of Beat the Menopause Without HRT *in my local bookshop, and decided to contact the Advisory Service for some personalised help.*

I had my first telephone consultation at the beginning of April 1996, and within six weeks of following the recommendations my flushes had greatly reduced and I was feeling more energetic. Unfortunately, in June of 1996 I discovered another lump in my remaining breast and, after careful thought, decided to have a second mastectomy.

I got through the operation with lots of family support and by August I was feeling brilliant. I was pleased to report to the WNAS that I had no remaining symptoms, and that I felt in control of my health. My husband is amazed and has even said I'm like a new woman. I am so pleased to be able to assume the role of a caring mum to three small children. I feel 100 per cent well – it's brilliant.

PHYTOESTROGENS AND OTHER HORMONE-RELATED CANCERS

The womb The endometrium, which is the lining of the womb, is particularly sensitive to oestrogens, and some of the risk factors for the development of cancer in this area are similar to those for breast cancer.

The cervix Cancer of the neck of the womb is closely connected with sexual activity, and is more likely to occur in women who had many sexual partners at a young age. There is now clear evidence that cervical cancer is associated with certain viruses that cause change in the cells covering the neck of the womb. The more prosperous individuals within a community, who probably have a better nutrient intake, seem to be at less risk of developing this type of cancer. Disturbed levels of nutrients have been detected in women with cervical cancer, but it not clear whether supplements of these would have any genuine protective effect at this stage. Irregular vaginal bleeding or bleeding after intercourse are two of the warning signs.

The ovary   Ovarian cancer is one of the most difficult cancers to detect and treat, which accounts for the fact that it claims more lives than many of the other types of cancer. Again, some of the risk factors are similar to those of breast cancer, including the family history aspect. Women with a family history of ovarian cancer should be screened regularly. Early detection, using ultrasound and blood tests, and subsequent removal of the ovaries would prove to be life-saving measures.

The general consensus from the wealth of studies that have been published on hormonally related cancer, indicate that in order to reduce drastically the chances of cancer we should be eating one serving of soya-based food per day, regular amounts of organic linseed, and as many other fruits, nuts, seeds, beans and berries as we can manage. Refer to the Phyto Products section, and suggested menus in Part Two for information and instructions.

The colon and rectum   Cancer of the large bowel may run in families, especially if the cancer developed at a young age, usually under the age of 45, and can also be associated with cancer of the womb, ovary or bladder. Colon cancer is more common in women, but cancer of the rectum claims more male victims. Those consuming a diet rich in meat and animal fat, and low in fibre and starch are more at risk. Low intakes of the mineral calcium are also thought to be associated with a higher risk of this type of cancer, or at least more rapid growth. Early detection by colonoscopy examination, X-rays and testing the stool for the presence of minute quantities of blood are all-important, and blood tests for detecting early tumours are currently being developed.

Once again, the research using phytoestrogens to prevent bowel cancer is showing very positive results. A Japanese study showed that eating soya beans or tofu cut the risk of rectal cancer by more than 80 per cent. Those who ate soya products had one-seventh of the risk compared to those who did not. Soya products also lowered colon cancer risk by about 40 per cent. In this particular study just one or two servings of soya per week gave considerable protection. Researchers in the USA have found that those who eat tofu regularly cut their risk of colon cancer by half. The Chinese confirmed these findings as they discovered that those who did not consume soya products on a regular basis were three times more likely to develop rectal cancer than the soya consumers.

Several studies have found that a high level of urinary lignan excretion, found in those eating a phytoestrogen rich diet, correlates with lower levels of colon cancer.

Recent research presented at the 3rd International Symposium on the Role of Soy in Preventing and Treating Chronic Disease concluded that subjects at risk of colon cancer who ate 39 grams of soya protein per day for one year had less cell proliferation in their colon and therefore reduced colon cancer risk compared with those in the control group who consumed 39 grams per day of casein. It concluded that eating soya may delay the onset of colon cancer and lead to more cancer-free years. Even if tumours develop while eating soya there are likely to be fewer, and they will grow more slowly.

Stomach cancer

One-third of Japanese Hawaiians consuming tofu were able to reduce their risk of contracting stomach cancer compared to non-consumers. In China, it was found that those who regularly consume soya milk had less than half the risk of developing cancer when compared to non-soya milk drinkers. In another Chinese study there was a 40 per cent reduction in the stomach cancer statistics in those consuming soya products on a regular basis. However, it should be pointed out that negative results have been produced when using miso. The probable reason for this is that miso, unlike many other soya products, is fermented and by nature rich in sodium (salt). As sodium is thought to be a risk factor for stomach cancer and possibly for other cancers as well, this may well be the reason for the increased risks with miso. On the positive side, it is thought that miso may protect us from radiation damage. Studies have shown that medical professionals tending atomic bomb victims did not develop tumours themselves because they regularly drank miso soup. Animal studies show that miso increases the radioactive discharge from the body. So perhaps miso should be included in the diet in moderation, unless you are at high risk for stomach cancer or have high blood pressure.

Prostate cancer

Like bowel problems, until recently prostate problems, particularly prostate cancer, was not a subject on the social agenda. It took the deaths of some eminent men, such as Frank Zappa, Telly Savalas and

François Mitterand, to increase public awareness about this potentially fatal condition. Nearly half of all men over the age of 50 develop an enlarged prostate, known as benign prostate hypertrophy, and prostate cancer kills four times as many men as cervical cancer kills women. The prostate gland is a reproductive gland that is wrapped around the urethra between the bladder and the penis. It is about the size and shape of a walnut, and is responsible for secreting the fluid that combines with sperm to form semen. Prostate symptoms include the frequent need to urinate, especially at night, and an inability to fully empty the bladder, sometimes leading to infection and pain with an erection or orgasm. Denis Norden, the presenter of 'It'll Be Alright on the Night', following his prostate operation, is reported to have said, 'When I was 20 my heart ruled my head. When I was 40 my head ruled my heart. But when I was 60 my bladder ruled both!'

Medication is used to treat prostate problems, and in some cases doctors resort to surgery. Natural remedies are also now widely available. Sabalin, a German product produced by Medic Herb, made from a herb called saw palmetto berries, has been through some very impressive clinical trials that showed a marked reduction in prostate symptoms. This product is distributed by Lichtwer Pharma and is widely available in healthfood shops and chemists and from the WNAS mail order service (see page 265).

Apart from skin cancer, cancer of the prostate is the most common form of cancer that men over the age of 55 are likely to experience. If caught in time it is treatable, and as some of the tumours are slow growing, the medical profession often carefully watches the progression rather than offering radical treatment. Screening tests are available in the form of a physical examination via the rectum, which can detect whether the prostate is enlarged, infected or whether there are any signs of a tumour. There are also prostate-specialist antigen blood tests available, and ultrasounds are often used before a diagnosis can be made.

Although Japanese men have the same prostate cancer rate as men in the West, they have the lowest death rate in the world from this particular cancer. As with other cancers, the growth of prostate cancer may be stimulated by hormones such as oestrogen and testosterone. Although oestrogen works in different ways in men, it can be equally destructive. Oestrogen, being a precursor to androgens, the male hormones, can trigger the production of testosterone, and studies have shown that men with prostate cancer seem to have higher levels of testosterone than their cancer-free counterparts. Once again phytoestrogens, particularly soya-based foods, seem to help moderate hormone levels, thus slowing down the growth of the tumour. Test-tube studies on genistein have shown growth of prostate tumour cells being inhibited.

A 20-year study of 8,000 men of Japanese ancestry living in Hawaii, showed that those who consumed tofu once a week or less were three times as likely to get prostate cancer as those who consumed tofu daily. It is interesting to note that Japanese men on average eat between 40 and 70 milligrams of genistein per day, compared to men on Western diets who eat in the region of one milligram or less. Another large study conducted on Adventist men, who have a high consumption of beans, lentils, peas and some dried fruits, which are all dietary sources of flavonoids, also have a much lower risk of prostate cancer. Conversely, a study performed by researchers at Harvard Medical School on 48,000 men, concluded that those who ate the most animal fat in the form of meat, butter, and chicken with skin, were at the greatest risk of developing more advanced prostate cancer.

Professor Herman Adlercreutz recently reported that in laboratory studies genistein and lignans (the fibre layers of grain, berries, seeds (linseeds), some vegetables and fruits), all inhibited prostate cancer cells to varying degrees. Studies on mice implanted with human prostate cancer cells who were fed rye bran and heated rye bran as well as soya had a slower onset of prostate cancer palpable tumours. Furthermore, the tumour volume was smaller. Rye bran also caused increased cancer cell death. He concluded that foods containing isoflavones and lignans may be protective with regard to prostate cancer.

Since prostate disease is considered to be sex-hormone dependent, an Australian study at Deakin University looked at the male sex-hormone responses in men after eating a tofu, lean meat or fatty meat meal. They found that sex hormone binding globulin (SHBG) significantly increased testosterone levels after both the tofu and lean meat meal, but not after the fatty meal. An increase in SHBG is considered positive as this helps 'mop up' excess testosterone, higher levels of which are a risk factor for prostate cancer. Lower levels of sex-hormone concentrations like testosterone may provide long-term benefits in reducing the risk of a disease like prostate cancer that appears to be sex-hormone dependent.

Lung cancer

Although lung cancer is often precipitated by cigarette smoke, active or passive, and to reduce your chances of becoming a victim it is advisable to live and work in a smoke-free environment, there is evidence to support the fact that once again certain phytoestrogens may help to protect us. A study of over 200 Chinese women in Hong

Kong found that by consuming soya products, including tofu, on a daily basis they were able to cut the risk of lung cancer by half, compared to women consuming soya products less than three times per month. Another Chinese study, this time on almost 1,500 men, found that the risk of lung cancer was reduced by 50 per cent with frequent tofu consumption.

Skin cancer

Although research in this important area is yet young, animal studies have been done to show that soya beans were able to delay the onset of skin tumours by 100 days and topically applied genistein reduced the number of skin cancers in mice.

The emphasis in *The Phyto Factor* is on prevention rather than cure. If, however, it is a cure you are looking for, there is certainly no harm in following the recommendations set out, whilst undergoing orthodox treatment. It is advisable to get your doctor's approval. Perhaps it would be an idea to take the book along to your appointment, in case your doctor is not familiar with the published medical references that are listed in chapter order at the end of the book. Part Two of this book concentrates on how the scientifically based dietary and lifestyle changes can be incorporated into your daily routine, with a view to keeping your cells healthy and free of cancer.

CANCER PREVENTION CHECKLIST

- Consume a diet rich in phytoestrogens, with a daily serving of soya-based food and as many other foods from the phytoestrogen list on page 66 as you can happily fit into your diet. Refer to the diet section in Part Two for sample menus
- Eat organically grown food when possible
- Limit your intake of fat, especially that of saturated animal fat, and use foods containing omega-3 and omega-6 essential fatty acids. See page 292 for the listings
- Do not smoke, and minimise your exposure to cigarette smoke
- Minimise your consumption of pickled and smoked foods
- Eat plenty of foods containing anti-oxidants, like fruits, vegetables and salad, particularly yellow vegetables like carrots and peppers, and green leafy vegetables. Aim to have at least five servings of fruit, vegetables and salad daily
- Take regular exercise and make time for relaxation
- Keep the stress in your life to a minimum

- Drink filtered or bottled water rather than water that contains chlorine
- Do not use pesticides or herbicides
- Minimise your use of Hormone Replacement Therapy and the oral contraceptive pill
- Use alternatives to plastic containers for storing food, and steer away from plastic products where possible as they release chlorinated toxins into the environment
- Purchase non-bleached paper, including writing paper, toilet tissue, coffee filters etc to avoid unacceptable dioxin exposure
- Use tampons and towels made without chlorine
- Avoid aerosols and anti-perspirants – use natural underarm deodorants
- Use hydrogen peroxide as an alternative to chlorine bleach for household chores, because it breaks down to water and oxygen.

11

PHYTOESTROGENS REDUCE HEART DISEASE

Coronary heart disease is now the most common cause of death in women in Western societies, with heart attacks claiming more than three times more lives than breast cancer and strokes more than twice as many. It actually accounts for 21 per cent of deaths of women over the age of 45 in the UK, and it is estimated that it costs the UK economy a total of around £10 billion each year. Women are protected from heart disease by the hormone oestrogen, prior to the menopause. Once they no longer are protected by oestrogen, the incidence of heart disease escalates post-menopause, so that women become far more at risk than men.

THE HEART

The heart is an amazingly strong muscular organ, which is tucked away in the left side of the chest wall. Its function is to pump blood through the arteries, in order to deliver fresh supplies of both oxygen and essential nutrients to all the organs in the body on a regular basis. Once the goodies have reached their destination, the blood pumped from the right side of the heart is pumped back, through the lungs, to dump the carbon dioxide it has collected and collect new supplies of reoxygenated blood. The refreshed blood returns to the left side of the heart, and is re-circulated through the body. Blood is prevented from flowing back in the wrong direction by a series of valves and chambers in both sides of the heart. On average, a human heart beats 100,000 times per day, amounting to over 3,000 million beats during the average female lifespan. The heartbeat you hear and the pulse that you feel is the regular pumping motion of the heart as it pumps the blood around the body. Like every other organ in the body, the heart needs a constant supply of oxygen and nutrients, which it takes, under normal circumstances, as the blood is passing through.

As the blood is pumped out of the heart into the arteries, it is at a higher pressure that the returning blood in the veins. When the heart contracts, the pressure rises to reach a peak called the systolic pressure, and between contractions the pressure falls off to what is termed the diastolic pressure. When you have your blood pressure measured, both these levels are recorded and are expressed as the systolic value over the diastolic value. It is well established that elevation of either levels can be associated with an increased risk of a stroke and other disorders of the circulation.

Blood pressure

Blood pressure values vary considerably from one person to another and from country to country. Even our own blood pressure picture varies during the course of the day, rising with stress, physical pain, exercise and sexual activity. There is usually a modest rise with age in urban populations, and until now this has been thought attributable to the relatively high intakes of sodium (salt) found in the diet of developed countries. In most developed countries, high blood pressure is measured as millimetres of mercury, which are written 'mm Hg', and anything greater that 140/90 is diagnosed as hypertension (high blood pressure) and worthy of investigation. For most adults, a rise in either diastolic or systolic readings above these values is associated with an increased risk of premature death.

HEART DISEASE CHECKLIST – ARE YOU AT RISK?

The heart disease questionnaire that follows is designed to give you some idea of your potential risk of having heart problems. It is only a guide and is not to be considered as accurate. Certain factors such as smoking, high blood pressure, diabetes, obesity and high blood cholesterol increase the risk. Exercise, eating fish, fruit and vegetables are associated with a lower risk. Family factors can be important, indeed anyone reading this book who has had a first degree relative (mother, father, sister or brother) experience a heart attack before the age of 55 should see their own GP for a more detailed assessment, no matter what their score on the questionnaire.

Fill in the questionnaire answering each question carefully and then add up your score. Some 'yes' answers score positively and some 'no' answers score positively, depending on the question.

HEART DISEASE QUESTIONNAIRE

	YES	NO
Do you smoke cigarettes?	3	0
If you are a non-smoker, have you smoked in the past 10 years?	1	0
Have you ever been diagnosed by a doctor as having heart disease or had a heart attack?	3	0
Has your mother, father, brother or sister had a heart attack or heart disease?	2	0
Are you a diabetic requiring insulin, diet or drugs?	1	0
If diabetic, have you had diabetes for more than 15 years?	1	0
Do you have high blood pressure needing treatment?	1	0
Is your blood pressure well controlled by treatment?	0	1
If you have had your cholesterol level checked was it:		
less than 5.2 millimols/litre?	0	
between 5.3 and 6.5 millimols/litre	1	
over 6.5 millimols/litre	2	
not tested	0	
What is your weight grade?		
2 or 3	1	
–1, 0, 1	0	
Do you exercise vigorously once or more per week or walk for more than 30 minutes per day, every day?	0	1
For women:		
Do you drink more than 3 units/day?	1	0
For men:		
Do you drink more than 5 units/day?	1	0
For men and women:		
Do you eat fish two or more times per week?	0	1
Do you eat fresh vegetables or fruit daily?	0	1

TOTAL SCORE _____

If your score is 0, 1 or 2 then this is a pretty low score and if there is no family history of heart troubles at an early age it would appear that you are less likely than average to have heart problems. A score of 3, 4 or 5 would suggest an average to slightly increased risk when compared with the rest of the population. If it is smoking, being overweight or lack of exercise that produced this score then it is obvious what you should do. Otherwise, see your doctor if you are not already receiving medical treatment. He or she can advise you about further risk factors and check your blood pressure and cholesterol if necessary.

If you scored 6 or over you must definitely check with your doctor, indeed it would be a good idea to see him or her before making a start on The Phyto Factor diet. Of course, if you already see your doctor because of high blood pressure or diabetes do discuss any points raised by this questionnaire that have not been covered by your treatment so far.

High blood pressure causes damage to the walls of the arteries, and the consequent risk to health is greatly magnified if an individual:

- Is overweight
- Smokes cigarettes
- Drinks alcohol excessively
- Has had an elevated blood cholesterol
- Eats a diet low in fresh fruit and vegetables and rich in animal protein
- Possibly has a poor intake of certain important nutrients, including vitamins C, E and magnesium.

Having mild or moderately high blood pressure often does not produce any symptoms at all, which is disturbing. Symptoms usually only occur when blood pressure is extremely high, and can include headaches, giddiness and a sensation of fullness in the head. Therefore, having a routine check-up from time to time becomes important.

« Jennifer Richie's Story »

Jennifer was a retired civil servant from Glasgow.

I approached the WNAS for help with my headaches and fatigue, which had become worse since taking HRT. I changed my diet as instructed, including foods that contained naturally occurring oestrogen, phytoestrogen-rich supplements, and began taking regular exercise and relaxation. Even after a few weeks I had so much more energy and my friends commented on how clear my skin looked. I'd been treated for high blood pressure and both my consultant and my GP were amazed to discover that since embarking on the WNAS programme my blood pressure had dropped into the normal range and my cholesterol level had reduced from 5.9 to 5.4.

When we enter the world, our arteries are clear and flexible, designed to contract and expand in order to accommodate the blood that is constantly being pumped around the body. As time progresses, if we mistreat our body, probably through ignorance, the arteries begin to narrow due to the gradual development of what is termed 'plaque'. This is made up of fatty deposits of cholesterol and fibrous tissue. Because of the plaque deposits, the internal diameter of the blood vessels becomes reduced; even small deposits of plaque can halve the blood flow through one of several coronary arteries. The process of arterial narrowing and hardening is called atherosclerosis. When plaque deposits have caused the arteries to narrow, the heart has to work harder to pump the blood around the body. Pressure builds up in the vessels, resulting in high blood pressure, which is a major risk factor for heart disease. When arteries supplying the heart itself become completely blocked the muscle in the portion of the heart that is denied both oxygen and nutrients will die, and the result is a heart attack. This process is known as ischaemic heart disease, and it causes 22 per cent of all female deaths in England and Wales, and 30 per cent of male deaths.

Heart disease past and present

Years ago heart disease was a rarity, probably associated with old age. These days, in the Western world heart disease has reached epidemic proportions, although numbers in recent years are starting to decline in countries like Australia, the USA and the UK, but they are still rising in Eastern Europe. The situation has become so dire that the beginning of atherosclerosis can even sometimes be detected in children. During the Korean War, researchers performed autopsies on nearly 2,000 American soldiers in order to study war wounds. They found more than they bargained for, as they discovered that three-quarters of these young men, with an average age of 22, already had the beginning stages of atherosclerosis. Women over the age of 50, post-menopause, generally suffer more with high blood pressure and heart disease than men, which is thought to be attributable to the fact that they are no longer protected by natural oestrogen.

This may sound very depressing, but considering the fact that although those living in the Western world are falling like flies, the majority of Asian communities generally reach old age with healthy blood vessels. We need to examine why this is so, and we don't need to look very far. During the Second World War, when food was rationed, there was a lack of meat and dairy products. Diets were largely based on vegetarian products like grains, vegetables and beans, which meant that the consumption of animal fat was low. During this time also, it just so happened that there was a dramatic decrease in heart disease.

THE CHOLESTEROL FACTOR

Cholesterol is a lipid, similar to fat, which has a waxy appearance. It is produced by the liver and can also be found in animal products. Cholesterol is needed by cells for energy, cell repair, the manufacture of vitamin D, sex hormones such as oestrogen and testosterone, as well as a number of other important functions. Because of its fatty nature it doesn't mix well with blood, which is mainly composed of water. It combines with protein in order to circulate in the bloodstream, and this combination is known as lipoprotein. High levels of cholesterol in the blood have long been associated with heart disease. In 1949 a study began of 5,000 men and women in Framingham, Massachusetts, and it is still ongoing today. The study was set up to determine the factors that are related to heart disease. Amongst many other things, they discovered that whilst no one in the study with cholesterol levels of less than 150 milligrams per decilitre (mg/dl) or 3.9 millimols per litre (mmol/l) had ever had a heart attack, the 50-year-old men, with blood cholesterol levels exceeding 295 (7.7 mmol/l) were nine times more likely to have a heart attack, compared to those whose cholesterol levels were around 200.

Whilst almost half of all Americans die of cardiovascular disease – approximately 4,000 citizens suffer heart attacks every day – a study in Shanghai, China, where the average cholesterol levels are in the region of 165 (4.3 mmol/l), showed only one in 15 dying of heart disease. According to Drs Brown and Goldstein, winners of the Nobel Prize for their work in cholesterol, desirable levels of cholesterol are between 100 (2.6 mmol/l) and 150 mg/dl (3.9 mmol/l), which is the level achieved by populations that consume low-fat, high-fibre diets. In the USA, it is estimated that 26 million American children have high cholesterol levels, and over 100 million adults have cholesterol levels that exceed 200 (5.2 mmol/l); half of those measure in excess of 240 (6.3 mmol/l), making a total of 52 per cent with high cholesterol levels. It is not a great deal better in Australia, where 47 per cent of men and 39 per cent of women have high blood cholesterol levels. The severity of the problem, however, increases with age, so by the time Australians are aged between 65 and 69, 62 per cent of men and 97 per cent of women have high blood cholesterol readings. In the UK the current average for women is about 28 per cent and 32 per cent for men.

Cholesterol – the good and the bad

There are two types of lipoprotein, the combination of cholesterol and protein, that flow around the body, which are quite different in

116

structure and function. The high-density lipoproteins (HDLs) are the 'good guys' and the low-density lipoproteins (LDLs) are the 'bad guys'. LDLs are designed to transport cholesterol to the body tissues, but too much LDL floating around the system will damage the arteries, and place you at greater risk of heart disease. The function of HDLs is to return cholesterol to the liver, in order for it to be broken down and excreted. They are even thought to help to prevent heart disease as they are capable of removing cholesterol from the artery walls and then carry it back to the liver for disposal. The ideal scenario is to have low levels of LDLs and higher levels of HDLs.

We do not actually need extra cholesterol from our diet, as the body is programmed to provide all the cholesterol that we actually need. However, when we consume a moderate amount of foods containing cholesterol, the body will compensate and make less natural cholesterol. When large amounts of dietary cholesterol are consumed on a regular basis, an overload situation occurs as both the liver and the intestines are programmed to continue to produce cholesterol no matter what. Dietary cholesterol is not present in vegetarian products, it can only be found in animal products. A portion of chicken with its skin on may contain much more saturated fat, but it contains precisely the same amount of dietary cholesterol as the equivalent chicken without its skin.

The deadly effects of saturated fats

Saturated fat is found in meat, dairy products, eggs, palm oil, coconut oil and chocolate; high intakes of these fats add to the risk of heart disease. The theory is that fat increases the production of the LDL cholesterol from the liver, which may then cause other blood changes, encouraging the depositing of cholesterol on the inner wall of the artery. Saturated fats are even more detrimental to cholesterol levels than dietary cholesterol itself, as they block the receptors in the liver whose function it is to remove LDL cholesterol from the bloodstream. One of the most famous dietary studies ever undertaken was a seven-country study conducted by Dr Ancel Keys. The findings confirmed that there was a direct relationship between the rate of heart disease and the amount of saturated fat consumed.

Other harmful ingredients in the diet, which raise blood cholesterol levels, are 'trans fatty acids', which form when vegetable oils are hydrogenated, in other words when hydrogen is added to them to make a solid fat. They are found in margarines that do not melt at room temperature, in cakes and biscuits, and are added to many processed foods. This means it is important to read the labels! Their effect on blood cholesterol is not as great as saturated fats, but they can by no means be considered desirable. In a large study published in the *The Lancet* in 1993, looking at women and coronary heart disease, Dr Willett and colleagues from Harvard University discovered that women consuming large amounts of trans fatty acids have a 50 per cent increased risk of heart disease when compared to women who consume little. Other statistics have suggested that the risk of these fats is small.

CAN DIET INFLUENCE GENETIC CHOLESTEROL LEVELS?

Many people who have genetically high levels of cholesterol are resigned either to living with the problem, or using drugs to control it. It is true that drug therapy can clear plaque from the artery walls and partially undo the damage that has been done, but it will only reduce the risks to a certain degree. The downside of long-term use of drugs is that they are expensive and not without side-effects. Following the widely accepted dietary recommendations to reduce fat intake by half, by avoiding animal fats and using lean cuts of meat, will also help to some degree, but is a regime that is still too rich in fat fully to reverse the problem. Another 'solution' to unblock clogged arteries is a procedure called angioplasty, where a balloon is inserted into the artery to widen it, or indeed to have bypass surgery. The problem that has emerged with these strategies is that, according to research, within ten years in some 40 per cent of the patients their original symptoms had recurred. Many scientists still feel we are stuck with the 'catch 22' of either settling for a restricted diet that only offers a partial solution, using expensive long-term medication, or resorting to surgery, which again has its limitations in the long term. However, a new and workable solution does seem to be emerging.

Almost 100 years ago it was discovered that animal protein, including meat, dairy products and eggs, could induce atherosclerosis. In 1990, researchers at the University of California confirmed that diet can be as effective at combating atherosclerosis as either drugs or surgery. The research team used a very low fat vegetarian diet, exercise and a meditation programme on a group of individuals with severely blocked arteries, which resulted in the arteries being cleared of plaque. Other fats such as oleic acid, found in olive oil and rapeseed oil, and polyunsaturated fatty acids derived from a variety of plant oils, fish oils and cold-pressed linseed oil, have the reverse effect. They actually shift the balance towards the good HDL cholesterol. The degree of protection that these 'healthy oils' provide is debated, and of interest not only to the general public and doctors, but also to farmers and politicians. The majority of expert recommendations in Western countries recognise a need for the 'average' consumer to reduce their total fat intake, by cutting down on saturated animal fats, maintaining a modest intake of polyunsaturates and making little change to the intake of oleic acid. No doubt the debates will continue for some time to come.

Many of the known risk factors also influence the balance between good HDL and bad LDL cholesterol. For example stopping smoking, correction of obesity and regular physical exercise may have a marked effect, reducing the total cholesterol and raising the ratio of good HDL to bad LDL. Unfortunately, doctors have not found it easy to raise HDL levels as they are largely determined by genetics. However, this is where soya and other phytoestrogens enter the picture.

The power of phytoestrogens

It was discovered almost by accident that soya protein lowers cholesterol levels. In the late 1960s researchers set out to find out whether soya could be a palatable alternative protein to meat, and in doing so they noticed a marked reduction in cholesterol levels in the soya consumers. Almost a decade later, soya was once again put under the microscope by Dr Sirtori at the University of Milan. He discovered that soya protein lowered cholesterol levels by an average of 14 per cent within two weeks, and by 21 per cent at the end of three weeks. Since that time, much more research has been undertaken to look at the effects of soya on cholesterol levels.

An analysis of 40 published studies was undertaken by Dr Kenneth Carrol at the University of Western Ontario. His conclusion was that 34 of the studies did produce a drop in LDL cholesterol levels in particular, by 15 per cent or more. Other more recent studies have shown that as well as reducing the level of LDL, soya has been successful in raising levels of HDL, the desirable cholesterol. Even genetically raised cholesterol levels have been seen to drop by 26 per cent in a four-week Italian study, published in 1991.

Another interesting study, conducted in 1999 by Dr John Eden from Sydney, Australia, showed that menopausal women on Novogen Red Clover supplements, containing 40 mg of isoflavones per tablet, showed an 18 per cent increase, on average, in HDL cholesterol.

A recent study by Professor Kenneth Setchell, reported at the 3rd International Symposium on the Role of Soy in Preventing and Treating Chronic Disease (Washington D.C., 1999) confirmed that it is possible to raise HDL, the good cholesterol, whilst lowering LDL, the bad cholesterol. His 12-week study, on 43 post-menopausal women consuming a soya-rich diet, containing 60–70 mg of total isoflavones each day, also highlighted the anti-oxidant effects of soya.

Futhermore, on 20th October 1999, the US Food and Drug Administration (FDA) approved a health claim for soya protein and its role in reducing the risk of coronary heart disease. This effectively means that food products that contain a minimum of 6.25 grams of soya protein per serving will be allowed to state on the label that in conjunction with a low-fat, low-cholesterol diet, the product may reduce the risk of heart disease. The health claim was developed by the FDA, which concluded, based on scientific evidence from more than 50 independent studies, that 25 grams of soya protein, included daily in a diet low in saturated fat and cholesterol, reduces the risk of coronary heart disease.

The Italians are so convinced about the value of soya in lowering cholesterol that it is now provided free of charge by the Italian National Health Service to those with high cholesterol levels. The benefits of phytoestrogens on lowering cholesterol levels and improving heart health are therefore an extremely important breakthrough in medicine.

Does this mean we switch to a vegetarian diet?

Those who enjoy their animal protein will be delighted to learn that research has also shown that it is possible to substitute some of the animal protein with soya, and still achieve highly acceptable results. Researchers from Sweden replaced half the animal protein with soya protein and managed to lower cholesterol levels by 25 per cent, and cutting meat intake in half caused a further drop of 10 per cent. Even replacing milk with a soya drink has resulted in lowered cholesterol levels. An American study has produced a 33 per cent drop in cholesterol levels within four weeks using just 20 grams of soya protein per day. And other American and Japanese workers have more recently replicated these finding using between 20 and 50 grams of soya protein per day.

HOW SOYA DOES IT

There are no firm conclusions about how this 'superfood' is able to reduce drastically the incidence of heart disease, but there are plenty of theories and hunches. According to information presented at the 3rd International Symposium on the Role of Soy in Preventing and Treating Chronic Disease, researchers are still trying to understand exactly how soya foods lower cholesterol. Studies where isoflavones are given on their own without soya protein in the form of a purified isoflavone pill, do not seen to lower cholesterol in humans. The current belief is that some amount of soya protein, or its non-isoflavone component, is necessary for the isoflavones themselves to be cholesterol lowering.

Let's examine some of the mechanisms that have been proven:

The amino acid factor   Compared to animal protein, soya has lower levels of essential amino acids, such as lysine and methionine, both of which have been shown to raise the level of LDL. It is also thought that the particular combination of amino acids found in soya may alter the composition of cholesterol.

The role of anti-oxidants   Soya has displayed its anti-oxidant properties in several studies, and it is believed by some that soya may reverse the oxidation of LDL by free radicals, thus preventing plaque formation. Recent studies have shown that soya protein and isoflavones can prolong the time taken before LDL cholesterol is oxidised. As it is the oxidised form of LDL which provides the raw ingredients for plaque, the less LDL oxidation, the better.

The binding factor   It has been suggested that soya may bind with bile in the intestines and then be excreted. This would necessitate the liver producing additional bile to compensate; to do this circulating cholesterol would be called upon, thus lowering cholesterol levels.

The blood pressure factor   In a study of peri-menopausal women, soya supplementation of 34 mg of isolated soya protein, given in a split dose throughout the day, reduced diastolic blood pressure by 5 mm of mercury.

The effect of oestrogen   It is well established that oestrogen lowers cholesterol levels, and it is thought that the phytoestrogen content of soya is able to perform the same task. Oestrogen plays a major role in the way lipids are produced, distributed and broken down.

The elastic artery promoting factor   Studies have demonstrated an improvement in arterial compliance associated with regular soya intake, meaning that the artery walls become more elastic. The less elastic and more constricted your arteries become, the harder your heart has to work to pump blood through the body, which can contribute to high blood pressure. Regular consumption of isoflavones will help to preserve the elasticity of your blood vessels and hence help to maintain a healthy heart.

The fibre factor   Soluble fibre, which is contained in foods like soya products, oat and rice bran and many fruits and vegetables, is acknowledged to reduce cholesterol levels. Because we cannot digest fibre, it passes into the colon where it is fermented by the local bacteria, a process thought to produce substances that may help to lower cholesterol levels.

The role of genistein This soya isoflavone seems to have the ability to inhibit the action of certain enzymes that promote plaque cell growth, thus reducing the amount of plaque formed in the narrowed artery walls.

The oestrogen receptors Whilst it has been known for some time that phytoestrogens are able to bind successfully to the oestrogen receptor sites within our cells, researchers have recently discovered a second oestrogen receptor, Oestrogen Receptor Beta, which is thought to play different roles in gene regulation. Oestrogen Receptor Beta sites are found in the brain, bone, bladder, lung, prostate, and our vascular tissues in particular, highlighting the selective action of oestrogens on different tissues.

The role of phytic acid Soya is a rich source of phytic acid, which is known to bind to iron, and may increase copper absorption in the body. It is thought by some that copper deficiency is related to high cholesterol levels.

Phytoestrogens as Selective Oestrogen Receptor Modulaters Phytoestrogens have certain similarities to 'designer hormones' (see section on SERMS, page 84), which are being developed to promote beneficial effects on the cardiovascular system and the skeleton, without having cancer-promoting effects on the breast and endometrium.

The thyroid function Those who have underactive thyroid glands tend also to have high levels of blood cholesterol. It is thought that soya may stimulate the thyroid gland to produce more thyroid hormone, thus reducing blood cholesterol levels.

There are a number of other components of soya, including lecithin, saponins and phytosterols that may help to reduce cholesterol levels. As research progresses, so too does the debate. The overwhelming conclusion, however, is that no matter how it does it, regular consumption of soya protein will genuinely help to lower high cholesterol levels. Additionally, those of us who do not suffer with elevated cholesterol levels can be confident that by adding soya to our diet, we are actively working to drastically reduce our risk of any future problems in the heart department.

SELF-HELP MEASURES

- Make sure you get proper medical care. Expert assessment and monitoring are required, but they are not always a foregone conclusion
- Consume a daily serving of soya
- Add organic linseeds to your breakfast cereal each day
- Lose weight, if you are overweight. Follow the Simple Weight Loss Diet, in *Every Woman's Health Guide*, or the *Zest for Life Plan*, for details refer to the Useful Reading list on page 257
- Don't smoke – it could mean the difference between life and death
- Reduce your animal fat consumption by at least half
- Eat three pieces of fresh fruit daily
- Consume two portions of green and yellow vegetables daily
- Include three portions of oily fish in your diet each week – mackerel, herring, pilchards, salmon or sardines
- Use mainly soya, linseed, rapeseed and walnut oils in your salad dressings
- Choose a polyunsaturated spread rather than butter
- Allow yourself one alcoholic drink per day – it appears that red wine in particular may be good for the heart
- Include in your diet garlic, onions and some nuts, including walnuts, almonds and pecans
- Regular exercise is a must, but you may need some specialised classes – get some advice from your doctor
- Consider taking nutritional supplements, as many are of proven value (see below)
- Avoid stressful situations both at home and at work
- Indulge in formal relaxation for at least 15–20 minutes each day.

The value of nutritional supplements

- **Nimostil**, a new product from Novogen, is a supplement containing formononetin. It has shown very encouraging results in clinical trials, benefiting both heart and bone health. Fifty post-menopausal women took the supplement for six months, and experienced on average a 28 per cent rise in their HDL levels, essentially restoring their HDL levels to pre-menopausal levels. This supplement is not available on the market as yet, but will undoubtedly be a useful addition on the shelves in the not too distant future.
- **Vitamin E** at high dose, 600 IU per day, has been shown recently to reduce the risk of a heart attack. A study of medical professionals showed that those who took a vitamin E supplement reduced their

123

risk of heart attack by 40 per cent. Take it, but don't think this means you don't have to do anything else. Those who are taking the blood-thinning drug warfarin will need to check with their doctor first, as vitamin E influences the effect of this drug.

- **Vitamin C** as a supplement of around one gram per day might help lower an elevated blood cholesterol, especially if you haven't been eating much fruit or vegetables.
- **Magnesium** might be helpful. Some studies have shown that very high doses help in the recovery from a heart attack. Additionally, magnesium deficiency has been shown to be common in those suffering with high blood pressure. Magnesium is likely to be needed by those who have low blood pressure levels as a result of taking diuretic (water) tablets.
- **Chromium** is a curious trace element. It is required in tiny quantities and helps insulin in its action of controlling blood sugar. Supplements have been shown to help correct a diabetic tendency and improve elevated blood cholesterol levels. Low levels of this mineral are associated with coronary artery disease. A supplement of 200 mcg per day is worth considering. It will need to be taken long term.
- **Multi-vitamins** are worth a mention. Perhaps the simplest thing to take is a modest strength multi-vitamin with vitamin E, 200 IU, and vitamin C, 250 mg. Older patients, those with a restricted diet, or those on many drugs may be the most suited to this.
- **Garlic** has had many positive studies on it – Kwai garlic has been shown to reduce blood cholesterol, increase blood fluidity, lower blood pressure and generally reduce the incidence of heart disease. The recommended dose is two tablets to be taken three times per day, with meals.

12

PHYTOESTROGENS AND THE PREVENTION OF OSTEOPOROSIS

Osteoporosis means 'porous bones', and is literally a condition that results in thinning of the bones. It has become an epidemic in the Western world, with an estimated five million sufferers in the UK alone. Every three minutes someone in the UK sustains a fracture due to osteoporosis. In Australians over 60 years of age more than 70,000 fractures are due to osteoporosis, and it is estimated that over 50 per cent of people with hip fractures will require long-term nursing care. Hip fractures claim more lives than cancer of the ovaries, cervix and uterus put together.

BONES

Our bones are composed of a 'skeleton' or scaffold of connective tissue around which minerals in crystalline form are laid down, rather like bricks being built up on a steel framework. The framework has a certain flexibility as well as great strength, and the minerals give the structure resistance to pressure or crushing, making the structure of bone rather similar to that of reinforced concrete.

During our lives, there is a constant turnover of bone. Until we reach the age of approximately 35, we lose as much old bone each year as we make new, hence keeping the scales in balance. From then on we tend to lose about 1 per cent of our bone mass each year until we reach the menopause, at which point bone loss accelerates with a further loss of 2 or 3 per cent per year for up to ten years.

In addition to the imbalance that develops in osteoporosis between bone loss and the rate at which new bone is deposited, there is also a reduction in the amount of connective tissue and the mineral content of the bone. The loss of bone mass reduces its strength and increases the likelihood that the bone will break when pressure is brought to bear on it.

As a result of osteoporosis, one in three women, and one in twelve men will suffer fractures of the hip, spine or wrist. Apart from the obvious pain and disability, osteoporosis often brings with it a loss of height and curvature of the spine, known in the UK as 'dowager's hump'. Within six months of sustaining a hip fracture, it is estimated that some 20 per cent of patients will die. However, what is not widely appreciated is that osteoporosis is both preventable and treatable.

ARE YOU AT RISK?

- Did you consume a poor diet, low in calcium, especially dairy products in your formative years?
- Do you regularly consume red meat and dairy products, rather than including vegetarian sources of protein in your diet?
- Did you experience an early menopause, spontaneously, or following surgery?
- Do you have a history of thyroid or other hormonal problems?
- Have you been underweight, or suffered any eating disorder such as anorexia or bulimia?
- Have you always had a petite build?
- Are you a smoker, smoking ten or more cigarettes per day?
- Have there been times in your life when you drank alcohol to excess regularly (more than the equivalent of 14 glasses of wine per week)?
- Do you take little formal weight-bearing exercise?
- Do you lead a sedentary lifestyle?
- Have you had periods of excessive physical activity in your life, e.g. have you been an athlete or a ballet dancer?
- Have you taken steroid drugs for an extended period of time?
- Have you suffered more than one fracture since your menopause?
- Has a close relative suffered with osteoporosis?
- Have you experienced a chronic illness which affected your digestion, kidney and liver function?
- Did you cease regular menstruation for a period of time, especially when you were young?

If you answered yes to any one of these questions, you have a higher than average risk of osteoporosis. If you answered yes to more than two questions, you need to take the subject very seriously, and certainly follow the recommendations in this chapter and the plan outlined in Part Two. It would be advisable to ask your doctor to refer you for a bone density scan, in order that you can assess together whether you need to address early osteoporosis, or merely follow a prevention campaign. I always recommend that our menopause and post-menopausal patients, who are not taking HRT, have a bone density scan repeated every three years, for peace of mind if nothing else.

Bone density

There are a number of dietary, lifestyle and environmental factors that influence the strength and density of bones. The mineral content of a woman's bones at the time of the menopause is not so much influenced by her current dietary intake as by her past intake of calcium over the previous 40 or 50 years.

WHAT DETERMINES THE STRENGTH OF OUR BONES?

- Diet, especially the intake of calcium during the growing years
- Physical activity, particularly weight-bearing exercise
- Hormonal factors, particularly the balance of oestrogen
- Genetic factors, which determine the size of bones and muscles
- Optimum levels of nutrients like calcium, magnesium, boron and essential fatty acids.

Our Western diet has much to do with the risks of developing osteoporosis in the same way as it influences heart disease and cancer. Many of us consume a diet which, though adequate in the short term, does not provide a good or optimum intake of nutrients and other dietary necessities in the longer term, thus predisposing us to diseases such as osteoporosis.

Calcium

Until recently, calcium intake was thought to be one of the most important factors in the prevention of osteoporosis. Average intakes in the UK for women are around 700 mg per day, the amount provided by just over one pint of milk, whereas recommended daily intake is at least 1000 mg per day in the UK and 1,200 mg per day in the USA. However, many consume less than this, and doing so during childhood and early adult life will mean that they reach middle and old age with a low bone mass and a high risk of osteoporosis.

On average, we carry approximately 1.3 kilos (3 lb) of calcium around with us, distributed roughly as 99 per cent to our bones and 1 per cent left circulating in our bloodstream. The blood calcium is necessary for many important functions including blood clotting, optimum muscle function and nerve transmission. When blood calcium becomes low, it is leached from our bones into the bloodstream; this is controlled by the hormone parathonmone secreted by the parathyroid gland. Up to two-thirds of our calcium intake may never reach our bones because of certain dietary or environmental factors. We know that common foods such as bran and tea are rich in phytates, and that phytates interfere with the absorption of calcium from our diet. (See the section on phytates on page 21.) This cannot be the total answer to the problem, for soya products are also rich in phytates and, as you will see, appear to minimise our risk of bone loss. A diet rich in salt and animal protein does appear to increase the loss of calcium from the urine, quite substantially.

Once we reach adulthood, no matter how much calcium we consume, it will not strengthen bones when they have stopped growing. However, the picture is not as gloomy as it may seem for there are many other aspects of our diet, which can dramatically reduce the rate at which we lose bone.

Calcium controversy

When the international statistics for osteoporosis are examined a contradiction becomes apparent, for some of the nations with the highest calcium intake also have the highest rates of osteoporosis. Conversely, those that have low intakes of calcium have some of the lowest rates. What confuses the issue even further is that, according to anthropologists, over 10,000 years ago, no humans other than infants were able to drink milk, for they lacked the enzyme lactase required to digest lactose (milk sugar). Hence, we open the door to an alternative underlying reason for the ever-escalating casualties created by osteoporosis.

Vitamin D

This is mainly derived from the action of sunlight on the skin and only small amounts come from the diet. It is needed to enhance the absorption of calcium from the diet. Levels are often low in the very elderly.

Essential fatty acids

Recent research suggests that the derivatives of the essential fatty acids (EFAs), GLA and EPA play a role in the absorption and metabolism of calcium, influencing the balance and amount of calcium in our bodies, especially in our bones. There are two types of essential fatty acids, the omega-3 series and the omega-6 series. The omega-3 series are derived from fish oils, oily fish including mackerel, herring, salmon, pilchards and sardines, as well as from some cooking oils such as rapeseed, soya beans, walnuts and golden linseeds (flaxseeds), which are the richest source of omega-3 essential fatty acids known. The omega-6 series of EFAs are found in evening primrose oil (EPO), sunflower oil, sesame oil and margarine made from them. Other good sources are eggs and turkey.

Magnesium

This mineral has come from obscurity to the verge of fame in the last ten years. It is the cousin of calcium and is necessary for normal bone, muscle and nerve function. In our work with women with premenstrual syndrome at the WNAS, we have repeatedly found that between 50 and 80 per cent of women whose blood levels we measured had low red cell magnesium. Not surprisingly, individuals with osteoporosis have also been shown to have abnormal bone magnesium levels. Despite this, over-the-counter or indeed prescribed supplements, rarely contain magnesium. Good sources of magnesium are unsalted nuts, wholegrains, green leafy vegetables and soya beans. There is a full list of magnesium-rich foods in the Nutritional Content of Foods list on page 285.

Boron

This is a trace mineral, found in fruits and vegetables, which appears to work in tandem with calcium and magnesium to build strong bones. It increases blood serum levels of oestrogen, and in turn oestrogen helps to maintain our bone levels of calcium and magnesium. It has a positive effect on calcium and active oestrogen levels in post-menopausal women. Supplementing the diet with 3 mg of boron daily has been shown to reduce urinary calcium excretion by 44 per cent and dramatically to increase the levels of the most biologically active form of oestrogen, oestradiol.

Animal fats

Another factor that emerges from the charts of international statistics relating to osteoporosis is that populations that have a high intake of animal protein are at greater risk of hip fractures through osteoporosis. Coincidentally, many of these nations are the very same countries that have a high calcium intake. Amongst scientific communities, this should not be a surprising finding, for as far back as 1930 researchers noticed that diet rich in animal protein resulted in heavy excretion of calcium through the urine. In the 1970s and 1980s, further research showed that there was a correlation between the amount of animal protein humans consume and the amount of calcium they subsequently lose through the urine. For example, an increase in protein from 48 grams per day, just below the recommended daily allowance, to 95 grams per day, which is close to the average daily consumption in the USA, resulted in 50 per cent more calcium being excreted through the urine. When protein intake was increased to 142 grams per day, even when the calcium intake was maintained at 1,400 mg per day, the individuals went into negative balance, meaning they were losing more calcium from the body than they were retaining. In another study conducted at the University of Texas Health Centre, different types of protein were used and calcium excretion through the urine measured. One group consumed meat and cheese, another had soya milk, textured vegetarian protein, cheese and eggs, and a third group consumed protein only from soya products. Even though each group consumed the same amount of protein and calcium in the diet, those in the meat and cheese group lost 50 per cent more calcium from their bodies than those in the soya group, and the loss of calcium from the combination group was somewhere in the middle.

In addition to this, smoking, alcohol, a poor diet and some conditions such as eczema and diabetes disturb the metabolism of these essential fats and can lead to deficiency states. It appears that a number of connected minor nutritional deficiencies have resulted in many of us being at increased risk of osteoporosis from middle age onwards.

Before we talk more about the role of phytoestrogens in bone health, let us look at oestrogen, as it is often prescribed by doctors to help maintain bone mass.

Oestrogen

An important part of oestrogen's role is to maintain bone mass and help with the constant process of bone remodelling. When oestrogen levels are optimum, bones are constantly regenerating, but when levels fall calcium is no longer directed to bones and the net result is bone loss. Bone mass is at its peak during the early thirties, and from then on it declines, with an annual bone loss rate of approximately 1 per cent per year.

Women who experience an early menopause, or who stop menstruating because of excessive dieting or exercise, have depressed levels of oestrogen and as a result are at greater risk of osteoporosis.

WHAT CONVENTIONAL MEDICINE HAS TO OFFER

Ordinary X-rays are used to detect existing fractures, but a measure of bone mineral density, using a specialised form of X-ray, is needed to measure bone mass and to monitor the results of treatment. Those with a high risk, or with established osteoporosis, should be scanned at regular intervals of between one and two years.

Simple blood and urine tests are being developed to help identify those who are likely to be 'fast bone losers'. The blood tests are for calcium and bone chemistry; blood and urine tests are for hormones.

There are a number of very different treatments available for those with osteoporosis. Your own doctor will need to assess which of these options is the most appropriate for you.

Hormone Replacement Therapy

The usage of HRT in the first ten or more years of the menopause is associated with a small, but significant reduction in the hip fracture rate in women. However, up to two-thirds of women who take HRT come off it within the first nine months because of side-effects or dissatisfaction. Although women taking HRT have a considerably greater bone mass than women who have not, this does not appear to be sustained in the longer term. After 20 years of taking HRT, it seems that there is a tailing-off effect, and the women who took HRT may only have a 3 per cent greater bone mass than women who, for their own reasons, did not take it.

For women who have an early menopause (before the late forties), and for some of the others in high-risk groups, it is probably advisable to discuss with your doctor the risks and benefits of taking HRT. Before doing so, read the section on the 'Pros and Cons of HRT', in Chapter 9. Those women who start the menopause after their late forties will be well-advised to help themselves to better bone health, certainly if they are unable or unwilling to tolerate HRT. Indeed, research shows that there are many tools which will help to preserve our own bone mass quite successfully.

OTHER MEDICAL TREATMENTS FOR OSTEOPOROSIS

Calcium supplements with Etidronate or Alendronate

Etidronate (Didronel PMO) and Alendronate (Fosamax) are synthetic compounds based on phosphorus, which combine with calcium in the bones and help to prevent its loss. They reduce bone loss in the spine and in the case of Fosamax, in the hip and the forearm. Fracture rates may also be reduced. These treatments are usually combined with calcium or a calcium-rich diet. They are available on prescription and need to be taken for a two-to-three-year period in order to reduce established osteoporosis. Unfortunately, they can produce side-effects, and usually can only be taken for a limited period.

Calcium supplements with vitamin D

These are a useful treatment for the very old and those with poor sunlight exposure. Low levels seem common in elderly Europeans, especially if they are housebound. Although vitamin D is necessary for the absorption of calcium from the diet, most of us synthesise enough from sunlight. Giving strong vitamin D supplements to those who are not deficient can actually cause bone loss due to excess stimulation of the bone-dissolving cells. Supplements containing vitamin D should therefore be taken with caution unless there is a proved deficiency.

Calcitonin

Calcitonin is a hormone produced by the thyroid gland and secreted when blood calcium rises. This is a hormonal treatment given by injection, which can be quite effective. This hormone influences the movement of calcium around the body. It is not a sex hormone. Its inconvenience limits its popularity.

THE ROLE OF PHYTOESTROGENS IN THE PREVENTION OF OSTEOPOROSIS

Japanese women have half the hip fracture rate of women in the West, and women in countries like Hong Kong and Singapore suffer even fewer fractures. One explanation could be that Asian women are more active. Japanese women, who traditionally sit on the floor, probably have stronger muscles and bones as a result of their regular movement, compared to a woman leading a sedentary lifestyle. But there is more to it than that, as new research is beginning to unveil.

We have already established that animal protein promotes calcium loss, and it seems soya protein has a protective effect. Animal studies have been conducted to compare the effect of premarin, a hormone replacement made from pregnant mares' urine, and genistein on bone health. The result showed that low-dose genistein was able to prevent bone loss almost as well as premarin. Dr John Anderson, at the University of North Carolina, who initiated the animal work, speculates that genistein's possible effects on bone may be due to its weak oestrogenic properties. Bone cells, like reproductive cells, have oestrogen receptor sites. At the time of the menopause, when oestrogen levels fall, the receptor sites in bones become redundant. It is likely that phytoestrogens continue the function of the natural oestrogen that was circulating around the body prior to the menopause, thus minimising bone loss.

A recent publication encompassed three animal studies in which researchers at the University of Western Australia set out to examine a potential role for phytoestrogens in post-menopausal bone loss. After six weeks the subjects receiving phytoestrogens had significantly reduced bone loss at all the sites that were measured.

Daidzein, another soya isoflavone, also seems to be providing good news on the bone front. A drug called Ipriflavone, which is made from daidzein, has been approved in Europe and Japan for the treatment of osteoporosis as it slows bone loss and stimulates the growth of new bone. It is being marketed as a pharmaceutical supplement at a dose of 600 mg per day.

Researchers are still trying to fathom why soya seems to be calcium sparing when compared to animal protein. One theory is that soya protein has low levels of the sulphur-containing amino acids, which cause the production of sulphate in the urine. Sulphate is known to work with the kidneys to prevent calcium from being reabsorbed into the bloodstream, and instead to be excreted through the urine. In addition to this, most high-protein foods contain phosphorus, which although it reduces the amount of calcium lost in the urine, increases the calcium loss in bowel motions. This may put regular meat eaters at an even greater disadvantage, as meat contains low levels of calcium, regardless.

The optimum regime for better bone health has to encompass all aspects of the research. We should of course include calcium in the diet, but at the same time reduce our intake of animal protein and increase our consumption of soya protein. It appears the calcium-only crusade may have backed the wrong horse, by treating osteoporosis as a deficiency disease. If it is a deficiency, it must be of oestrogen, rather than of calcium.

SELF-HELP MEASURES

Do not underestimate the benefits of self-help measures. Each of the diet and lifestyle changes will, by themselves, make little difference in the short term, but over a period of years are likely to be of substantial benefit. Many of the measures will help not only osteoporosis, but will also help to reduce the risk of heart disease and stroke.

« Jane's Story »

Jane Harrison was a 48-year-old mother of three from Folkestone in Kent, who had been suffering with her symptoms for two years when she sought help from the WNAS.

I served in the police force for many years, and was five feet, five inches tall on my inception. Following a prolapse I had a hysterectomy five years ago, and although my ovaries were intact, my doctor prescribed HRT in the form of Premarin.

I persevered with the HRT for a few years, but was put off by the awful side-effects of nausea, depression and weight gain. I put on 16 lb which took me from a trim size 12 to a large size 14. I was afraid to stop taking the HRT as I noticed from comparing height with other family members that I had lost two inches. Additionally I knew that my mother had lost six inches off her height and my father had osteoporosis after long-term use of steroids.

I eventually came off the HRT two years ago because I felt so awful and the night sweats and flushes that followed were flattening. My skin became very dry and the condition of my hair had deteriorated. One year later I read a magazine article about the Women's Nutritional Advisory Service's holistic approach to the menopause and, as the case history in the article sounded just like me, I decided to book an appointment at their clinic.

During my consultation, a programme of diet, exercise, relaxation and nutritional supplements was worked out, and I got started straight away. I adjusted to the programme quite quickly and soon noticed that I was feeling better in myself.

Within two months the flushes calmed down, my libido started to return, and I generally felt more positive.

A year on I have gone from strength to strength. I feel well, I no longer suffer with symptoms of the menopause, and the condition of my skin and hair has improved. I have continued to take the multivitamins and the Efacal the WNAS suggested and am managing my health myself.

I never did have a bone density scan so I have nothing to compare, but I haven't lost any more height and I feel more agile than I have for years.

DIETARY AND LIFESTYLE TIPS

- If you are around the time of the menopause and beyond, consume foods that contain phytoestrogens daily. Refer to the Phyto Products list on page 250, and follow the suggested menus and recipes in Part Two.

- Make sure your diet contains a variety of foods rich in essential fatty acids. See page 292.
- Concentrate on eating nutritious foods that are also rich in calcium and magnesium – see the lists commencing on page 291.
- Consume foods rich in vitamin D if you do not get much sunlight exposure. They include dairy products, margarine, semi-skimmed milk, eggs, or fortified cereals like cornflakes and Rice Krispies.
- Avoid excessive consumption of sugar and foods rich in sugar such as fizzy drinks, sweets, cakes and biscuits.
- Reduce your intake of salt, both added to cooking and at the table and avoid salty foods like bacon and kippers.
- Eat vegetables and salads daily.
- Eat at least two servings of fresh fruit per day.
- Limit your intake of saturated animal fats by consuming leaner cuts of meat and reduced fat dairy products, and by avoiding fried foods. This is particularly relevant if you are overweight.
- Reduce your intake of tea, coffee, cola and chocolate, which all contain caffeine.
- Limit your consumption of alcohol to a maximum of three to four drinks each week. One unit of alcohol is equivalent to one glass of wine or $1/2$ pint of beer or lager or one spirit, sherry or vermouth. Women who stop smoking and drinking at the time of the menopause may reduce their hip fracture rate by as much as 40 per cent.
- If you smoke, try to cut down gradually or, better still, give up altogether.
- Both smoking and drinking alcohol have a broad spectrum anti-nutrient effect and accelerate the loss of nutrients. In addition, smokers and those consuming excessive amounts of alcohol usually have different diets and different essential fatty acid levels too, but it's never too late to stop!
- Take a supplement rich in calcium, magnesium and boron, with supplements of marine fish oil and evening primrose oil. These help to increase the uptake of calcium across the gut wall and reduce the loss through the urine. In addition, consider taking one of the phytoestrogen supplements listed on pages 68–71.
- See your doctor if you are a high risk case, to discuss assessment and other treatments.

EXERCISE

Exercise is a valuable tool at all stages of life to promote good health. It is an acknowledged way of helping to protect against heart disease and to help keep bones strong. At the time of the menopause, when women are most at risk of bone loss, exercise must become a vital part of the everyday schedule. Any combination of the following suggestions are acceptable:

• jogging	• skipping
• brisk walking	• dancing
• playing racquet sports	• press ups
• lifting weights	• squeezing tennis balls
• workouts	

Research has shown that weight-bearing exercise, in other words anything that involves putting pressure on your bones, helps to stimulate the regeneration of bone tissue by reducing calcium loss.

The consensus from studies is that you need to exercise moderately three or five times each week, for 30–45 minutes each time, so long as you do not suffer with cardiovascular disease. The pay-off, apart from helping to strengthen your bones, will be that within 12 weeks you can expect to feel more energetic, cope with stress more effectively, sleep better, have increased resistance to infection and feel a lot better generally!

The disabled, the bedbound – even if it is only for a few weeks – and the housebound are very much at risk, as are astronauts because of the weightlessness.

However, bear in mind that too much exercise can be damaging. It is now known that young female athletes, gymnasts and ballet dancers are high-risk groups for osteoporosis. Their intensive training and low body weight often prevent them from menstruating, resulting in lowered levels of oestrogen, which subsequently affects their bone mass.

It is important that those who exercise vigorously have an adequate and nutritious diet in order to maintain their body weight. Failure to do so will further increase the risk of osteoporosis.

I know there is a long list of factors to consider and actions to take, but it is important that no stone is left unturned, as we only have one set of bones. As you can see, there is a great deal we can do to help ourselves to better bone health.

13

PHYTOESTROGENS IN THE MANAGEMENT OF DIABETES

DIABETES

Diabetes mellitus, as it is properly known, is a condition in which there is a chronic rise in the level of glucose in the blood, which routinely spills out into the urine. The word diabetes means 'a flowing through, or siphon' and mellitus means 'sweet'. Urine is frequently passed because the high level of sugar pulls water along with it. Other characteristics of diabetes are increased thirst, a craving for sweet foods and fatigue due to the effect the increased sugar has upon the body's metabolism. Other symptoms may include changes in visual acuity, recurrent thrush, muscle cramps, tingling in the feet and hands and constipation.

Diabetes is an exceedingly common condition, particularly in Western countries. It is estimated that between one-third and one-half of all diabetics in the world live in America, which amounts to between 5 and 10 per cent of their population, and surprisingly half of them don't even know they have it. The cost of diabetes in the USA is $91.8 billion, with 798,000 new cases annually. In Australia, diabetes is likely to affect 900,000 citizens by the year 2000, and 1.15 million by the year 2010. Australia has a very high rate of insulin-dependent diabetes compared with the rest of the world, and the cost to the nation exceeds $1 billion annually. In New Zealand diabetes costs the nation $450 million annually, just over 10 per cent of the national budget. And in the UK in the mid-1990s, diabetic illness consumed 5 per cent of the total £29 billion budget.

Whilst 50 per cent of some populations around the world become victims of diabetes, in many parts of the world diabetes is rare. In Third World countries, where people have just enough food to survive and are continually undertaking physical tasks, diabetes is hardly an issue, and in richer countries, during the World Wars when food was in short supply, the number of new diabetics reduced dramatically. This clearly demonstrates that the incidence of diabetes is related to diet.

The function of insulins

Our blood glucose levels are controlled by what we eat, a variety of hormones and by the function of the liver and muscles. In medicine, there is a wide variety of situations, many of which are rare, where blood glucose control is disturbed. Understandably, this happens with liver and muscle disorders and a number of exotic hormonal conditions, as well as in some pregnancies. The most important hormone in blood glucose control is insulin, which is produced by the pancreas, a gland situated in the abdomen. The role of insulin is to help glucose pass from the bloodstream into cells, especially of the nervous system, muscles and the liver. To all these organs glucose is a source of energy, and uniquely for the nervous system it is the only source of energy that it can use. When a person becomes diabetic, their cells can no longer get the glucose they need in order to survive. Under normal circumstances, cells derive glucose from complex carbohydrates in the diet, which are broken down into glucose during the digestive process and then absorbed into the bloodstream for transportation to the cells. One of the functions of the hormone insulin is to take glucose to the receptor sites in the surface of the cells, which recognise insulin and allow it to enter.

Diabetes used simply to be divided into two main types – insulin-dependent (IDDM) Type I and non-insulin-dependent (NIDDM) Type II. In the insulin-dependent variety there is a lack of the hormone, which must then be given by injection. In the non-insulin dependent form there is plenty of insulin circulating in the bloodstream, but the tissues of the body are relatively insensitive to it. The cells of a Type II diabetic effectively lose their memory and no longer recognise insulin, which means that much of it is left circulating in the blood and eventually is excreted in the urine. In the absence of insulin the cells literally starve. This type does not need insulin, but a diet and drugs that improve the uptake of insulin by the cells.

Insulin is an extremely important hormone with many functions. It plays an active role in the growth of cells, the production of new proteins and fat metabolism. There is now a more complicated classification of diabetes, based upon not only the need for insulin, but also the probable cause or causes of that type of diabetes.

What causes diabetes?

This is one of the great questions of twentieth-century medicine and it is being answered in a curiously piecemeal way. The pieces of the jigsaw include:

- Genetic factors, which are particularly important for the insulin-dependent diabetic. It is predominantly a disease of Caucasians, but not exclusively from the northern part of Europe. There are many environmental factors too: if members of a low-risk population, such as the Japanese, emigrate to a high-risk country like the USA, their risk pattern follows that of US residents.
- Genetic factors for the non-insulin-dependent diabetic. Usually, the adult onset form of diabetes, which seems to run in the female line of the family, may be linked with other conditions affecting muscles. It may also be linked to those with a tendency to high blood pressure and raised blood fats.
- Immune changes which cause the body to produce antibodies that attack the insulin-producing beta cells of the pancreas. This may be genetically determined and triggered by some viral infections.
- Food allergy. This is a possibility, as some researchers report that the antibodies involved in cow's milk allergy can also react against the pancreas. This seems particularly relevant to children.
- Being overweight. This is an extremely important risk factor, especially for the elderly with NIDDM. People with Type II diabetes are often considerably overweight, with surplus fat in the tummy area, rather than on their hips and thighs.
- Being small at birth. This has also been shown to be a risk factor, perhaps reflecting a reduced ability to produce insulin in a better form that is functional. This risk does not appear until later life, and can become marked if the individual is obese, has high blood pressure and elevated blood fats.
- Diseases where the pancreas is damaged or destroyed.
- Various types of malnutrition in Third World countries.
- A number of other hormonal problems affecting the adrenal glands or the ovaries.
- Rare genetic disorders.
- Following drug therapy, especially thiazide diuretics, if deficient in potassium.
- Pregnancy, resulting in a large baby.

This is a fantastically diverse list. In practice, for the majority of those with, or at risk of developing diabetes, dietary factors are the most important area that we can do something about on an individual level.

Apart from the fact that diabetes is life threatening in itself, diabetics are much more prone to high levels of cholesterol and to develop atherosclerosis. It can also cause damage to other parts of the body, including the nerves, kidneys, eyes, limbs and reproductive system, often causing impotence in men.

DIABETES AND DIET

Dietary modifications have been used to treat and control diabetes for centuries. A high carbohydrate diet was advocated by the early Egyptian doctors and this was later refined by the Greeks. However, by the end of the eighteenth century doctors had decided that carbohydrates, rather than helping diabetics, were detrimental to them. These views persisted until well into the twentieth century, when it was discovered by health professionals that populations eating a diet of predominantly plant-based foods, most of which are complex carbohydrates and low in animal fat, had much less diabetes.

A low-fat diet is essential for diabetics as they are more prone to atherosclerosis and obesity, and fat has been shown to upset blood sugar control. A study that was conducted at the Pritikin Longevity Center in California found that diet which contained only 10 per cent fat greatly improved Type II diabetes.

In 1917, John Harvey Kellogg wrote about the role of the soya bean in the control of diabetes. At about the same time two researchers with an interest in soya beans published a paper in the *American Journal of Medical Science*, which outlined how diabetic patients who consumed soya beans regularly, passed less sugar in their urine; a marker for the control of diabetes. There has been more recent interest in the role of soya fibre and the control of diabetes, as this fibre, which helps to control cholesterol levels, also seems to be able to regulate glucose levels and helps with insulin sensitivity. The high-fibre diet, consisting of oats, fruit, vegetables, and legumes including soya, appears to help the cells of the Type II diabetic recognise insulin, and thus allow entry into the cell.

In 1987, a study published in the *American Journal of Clinical Nutrition* compared using 10 grams of soya fibre at one meal, and then none at another sitting of the same meal. It discovered that when soya was included in the diet the blood glucose levels rose and fell at normal rates, compared to the non soya sittings where blood glucose rose to higher than normal levels and stayed there for longer than usual periods. Another study used just 7 grams of soya and compared it to cellulose, the insoluble fibre found in wheat bran and vegetables. For the three hours following the meal, the soya consumers had notably lower levels of glucose in their bloodstream compared to those who had consumed cellulose.

Furthermore, it seems that not only does soya have benefits for blood sugar control and heart health, but for kidney health as well. This is very important for people with diabetes, since nearly one-third of them develop renal disease. Diabetic renal disease (nephropathy) is a major contributor to death in those with diabetes. Nephropathy is damage to the tiny nephrons in the kidney, which act like minute filters. As a result of this damage, protein is filtered into the urine instead of being reabsorbed back into the bloodstream. This is a condition called microalbuminuria. The likelihood of nephropathy increases dramatically after having diabetes for ten or more years. The early stages of nephropathy are marked by an increase in protein leaking into the urine and an increased workload on the kidneys. Too much dietary protein can cause a faster decline in kidney function. However, it seems that not all proteins are created equal, as recent research suggests that soya protein may be protective for kidney health.

Research by the University of Kentucky presented at the 3rd International Symposium on the Role of Soy in Preventing and Treating Chronic Disease (Washington D.C., 1999) showed that changes in blood flow to the kidney following various protein meals was found to be greatest with beef, followed by poultry and fish. Soya protein does not significantly alter kidney function following a meal, which is good news. Other work by Professor Anderson in a group of six patients with Type I diabetes, who have early signs of kidney damage, shows that soy may help to conserve kidney health. Patients ate 55 grams of soya protein per day via a soya patty, soya beverage and soya pasta for eight weeks, then resumed their normal animal protein intake. After eating soya protein for eight weeks, these patients showed evidence of a decreased workload on their kidneys compared with when they were eating a normal diet. Two patients who were previously losing protein in their urine also lowered the amount lost after the eight weeks of soya protein. Also, the average reduction in total cholesterol and LDL ('bad' cholesterol) was 7 per cent and 13 per cent respectively. This is a highly positive outcome in reducing the risk of further health problems such as heart disease. This small study suggests that soya may be preventative for the early stages of diabetes, as well as having benefits for heart health.

« Sally's Story »

Sally is a 24-year-old waitress who has been diabetic since puberty. She has also had a history of repeated viral infections, including meningitis and shingles, and there was a strong suspicion that a virus infection had triggered her diabetes. Once, before attending the clinic, she had another viral infection that was just a bout of flu, which left her feeling very tired indeed, so that she had to give up work. Her diabetic control had deteriorated and she had made several attempts to improve this by adjusting her dose of insulin.

Her fatigue every day was quite severe, with muscular aches and pains, and the diabetic specialist discovered that the sodium level in her blood was very low. Investigations also revealed low levels of many other nutrients, especially magnesium, zinc and vitamin B.

She made some changes to her diet, took supplements of all these nutrients, except for sodium, and also took a multi-vitamin preparation. Her energy level duly improved, as did her diabetic control. Low levels of magnesium are common in diabetes and may influence the balance of other minerals, especially sodium and potassium.

SELF-HELP MEASURES

- **Learn about your diabetes** Join the British Diabetic Association (BDA). Be a professional patient.
- **Monitor your diabetes** This means regular, usually daily, tests of blood sugar for all those with IDDM, urine tests of sugar and sometimes protein. The intention is to keep the blood sugar level between 4 and 9 millimols per litre, though this may vary from person to person. There should be no glucose in the urine if kidney function is normal.
- **Be strict with your diet** Some parts of the diet described below may take some getting used to. The high intake of beans may cause an increase in abdominal wind and bloating. Be patient, this should settle after two or three months.
- **Exercise regularly** This helps keep weight down, reduces blood cholesterol, lowers blood pressure and may improve blood glucose control. The minimum is to walk for 30 minutes four times per week.
- **Don't smoke**
- **Limit alcohol intake** This should be kept to an average of no more than 2 units per day, with up to 4 units on special occasions.
- **Be aware of hypoglycaemia** This is low blood sugar and could be dangerous! Symptoms include light-headedness, confusion, anxiety, palpitations, hunger, shortness of breath and sweating. Unfortunately, some diabetics have little warning of these episodes and loss of consciousness develops quickly. Awareness is very important if they are driving or in charge of machinery.
- **Take some nutritional supplements** This is a very difficult, but potentially important area. Many small reports associate diabetes

with a lack of essential nutrients; most common if diabetes has been present for many years, if there is a poor response to insulin, and in older diabetics or those with complications. The lack of nutrients may not be corrected by a standard diabetic diet. Potentially important nutrients are:

- Vitamin B1 – thiamine is needed to metabolise glucose. Those first beginning on oral medication, alcohol consumers and the elderly are at risk. Fatigue, muscle pains in the legs and loss of feeling in the hands and feet are early symptoms.
- Magnesium – lack may develop with vitamin B1 deficiency, especially if the diet is poor. Lack of response to insulin and increased risk of damage to the blood vessels at the back of the eye can be features of a deficiency of this nutrient.
- Chromium – this is a curious trace element worthy of a particular mention in diabetes. It is involved in influencing the tissues' response to insulin, which is clearly important in the elderly diabetic with NIDDM. So much so that marked chromium deficiency produces a state virtually indistinguishable from this type of diabetes and is also associated with an increased risk of cardiovascular disease. Potentially, correcting a deficiency of this trace mineral could be beneficial to many diabetics. We will have to wait for more research to be performed to be certain about the role of chromium.
- Zinc – this is easily lost in the urine in diabetics. Poor resistance to infection, poor wound healing and possibly reduced response to insulin may be a feature.
- Vitamin B6 – pyridoxine has been used successfully to help control the diabetes that develops in pregnancy.
- Anti-oxidants – these include vitamins E, C, A, as beta-carotene, and selenium, and they are all involved in minimising the damage to tissues that occurs as part of ageing or with an altered metabolism. They may prove to be important in the progress of vascular disease, heart disease and cataract formation in the diabetic.
- Polyunsaturated fatty acids – these are essential nutrients and high intakes of the omega-6 series from vegetable oils reduces the risk of developing problems with the blood vessels at the back of the eyes. Specialised forms of these fats, such as evening primrose oil, have been used with a little success when the nerves are damaged by diabetes. Fish oils might be beneficial too, in reducing blood stickiness, but there could be problems with this.

Expert advice and individual assessment seems the best way forward until there are large and long-term trials to assess the benefits of using these types of supplements. It should be remembered that they are no substitute for good dietary control and, where necessary, insulin and drug treatment.

Important note
Do not take vitamin and mineral supplements, except perhaps for low-dose preparations, without the permission of your doctor. At times their use could alter insulin requirements and blood glucose control. Hypoglycaemia, a low blood glucose, could occur as a result.

Self-help advice on diet

This has assumed increased importance over the years. It is clear that control of blood glucose and the risk of serious and less serious complications are to a large degree influenced by the diet. The standard recommendations are as follows:

- Eat an appropriate amount of calories to achieve a reasonable weight; for most NIDDM patients this will mean losing weight. This may well be all that is required to normalise blood glucose levels.
- Eat regularly; consume three meals a day and where necessary snack between meals. Snacks are likely to be needed by children, those who are physically active and pregnant women, provided they are not overweight.
- The diet should contain a large amount of foods that are slowly digested and therefore cause only a small rise in blood sugar. This means excluding or severely limiting the consumption of simple carbohydrates – sugar, cakes, biscuits, white and, to a lesser extent, wholemeal bread. Desirable foods are fibre-rich complex carbohydrates and include beans, peas, lentils, pasta, oats and oat products, whole-wheat cereals, sweetcorn, soya products and most fruits.
- High-fat foods are to be limited. Intake of saturated fats in particular should be curbed. This means consuming low-fat dairy products including low-fat cheeses, trimming all visible fat from meat before cooking (by grilling or baking), not eating the skin of poultry and fish and not eating fried foods.
- The diet should be rich in polyunsaturates, e.g. sunflower, safflower, corn and soya oil. Olive oil can be used in small amounts, as can walnut oil. Butter should not normally be used and margarines high in polyunsaturates should be used in its place.
- High cholesterol foods should also be limited, especially if the blood fats are high. Up to eight eggs per week can be consumed.

- Ensure a regular intake of phytoestrogens in your diet in the form of soya products such as milk and tofu, and pulses, cereals and seeds. Refer to Chapter 7 on page 55.
- Further dietary advice may well be needed for those with heart or kidney disease, or who are pregnant, or for those whose diabetes is particularly difficult to control.

It is vital that your progress is monitored. Regular attendance at a clinic, either at your general practitioners or at the local hospital, will allow the early identification of problems and their treatment. Now let us look at the effect that our lifestyle has on our health.

14

LIFESTYLE AND OUR HEALTH PROSPECTS

We have examined the power of diet in relation to our health, but that is not the whole story, for our lifestyle and the environment in which we live play an enormous part in our well-being.

EXERCISE

Both weight-bearing and aerobic exercise have been shown to:

- protect your heart against heart disease
- influence your mood positively, decreasing symptoms of depression
- increase energy levels
- raise HDL cholesterol levels, which are the 'good' cholesterol levels discussed in Chapter 11
- burn excess fat, helping to maintain optimum weight and shape
- preserve your bone mass and help to prevent the bone-thinning disease, osteoporosis
- help to prevent constipation
- reduce levels of stress

If you are not already exercising regularly, you will need to work out a programme for yourself that consists of four or five sessions per week, to the point of breathlessness. It may only take a few minutes initially to get out of breath, but after a few weeks you should be exercising comfortably for 30 minutes at each session. Once you begin to feel the benefits of exercise, that will be all the motivation you need to keep you going.

The purpose of exercise

The object of exercise is to keep you fit and to speed up your metabolic rate. A considerable amount of research has been carried out on exercise in relation to health, and the conclusions are positively in favour of regular exercise. It does not matter what kind you undertake, as long as you adhere to two rules: you must enjoy the exercise you choose, and you should undertake weight-bearing exercise that is also aerobic.

Exercise time should be enjoyable, and not regarded as a competition. The only person you will be competing against is yourself, so if you haven't exercised for a while, ease into it gently. Go for brisk walks to start with, and don't over do it. It is far better to build up your stamina over a period of weeks, rather than to end up with muscular aches and fatigue. If you have any current health problems you should check with your doctor before you embark on an exercise programme.

Types of aerobic exercise

The types of aerobic exercise you can choose may vary from brisk walking, jogging, skipping, dancing, workouts, and racquet sports like squash and tennis to swimming and cycling. Those with a busy lifestyle, who find it too difficult to get to the gym or to an exercise class regularly, should perhaps invest in an exercise video to use at home. Although it may require more self-discipline than exercising with a partner or attending a class, it is a convenient way to get started and to build up your stamina gradually without embarrassment. You will need to set aside a regular time to exercise that fits in with your lifestyle. I find that exercising first thing in the morning works best for me, mainly because my days are so demanding and my evenings are full of family demands. Whatever schedule you select for yourself you must vow to stick to it, no matter what. It is all too easy to let your exercise routine slip, and watch your hard-earned fitness level evaporate within the space of three or four weeks.

THE IMPORTANCE OF RELAXATION

There is plenty of hard evidence to suggest that stress underlies many major health problems, and that regular exercise and relaxation are two sound ways of avoiding illness and keeping both your mind and body in good shape. Taking time out for yourself is not just a nice idea, it is a necessity, especially if you lead a full and demanding life. Stress can have a powerful effect on the body. It has been shown to suppress ovulation in menstruating women, to contribute to digestive disorders like irritable bowel syndrome, to play a key part in migraine headaches, and to increase the number and severity of hot flushes at the time of the menopause.

The stress factor

There is a fine line between stress and distress. Stress is reasonably healthy, as it stretches us to capacity and keeps us on our toes. Dealing with challenges as they present themselves is good for morale, but when we get to the point of overload we cross the line and our modern-day lifestyle often leaves many of us reeling, feeling overwhelmed and under par. If these symptoms continue for more than a short period of time our health can suffer.

Relaxation tips

- Make time each day to relax formally – you will need 15 or 20 minutes, with no interruptions. Take the telephone off the hook, inform those at home that it is your relaxation time, and either practise yoga, meditation, or my favourite, which is creative visualisation. You simply lie on the floor with a pillow under your head, do a bit of deep relaxed breathing, and then imagine you are somewhere exotic, doing whatever you find therapeutic. Really switching off is an art, and you may need some instruction or to read a book on the subject (see page 258).
- Get your partner or a close friend to give you a massage, preferably using some relaxing aromatherapy oils like geranium or lavender mixed with a base oil like sweet almond.
- Watch an entertaining film or make time to read a good book.
- Make sure you laugh occasionally. Laughter is so good for us, and yet when we get absorbed with problems in life we seem to lose our sense of humour.
- Hum in the bath, as it has been shown to improve your mood and energy levels!

CLEANING UP THE ENVIRONMENT

Much of the food we consume has been subjected to chemicals at some point in the food chain. Many foods contain chemical additives in the form of flavour enhancers, colouring and preservatives. While some of these are not harmful, some of them are and our bodies are certainly not designed to cope with them. These days meat animals are bombarded with antibiotics, to the point where they often become resistant to them. They are used as a preventative measure and often used for growth promotion. Nitrate fertilisers have been used to obtain fast-growing and abundant crops, but it is now recognised that nitrates are harmful and can produce cancer, at least in animals. Almost all fresh fruit, cereals and vegetables are sprayed with pesticides at least once. In addition, milk and meat may retain pesticides from feed given to live-stock (see page 26 for details about how chemicals in milk affected women in Israel).

All these processes in the rearing and growing of food mean a reduc-tion in basic nutrition. One solution that is within our control is to buy organic foods, which have not been exposed to chemicals. Although organic food is harder to obtain (unless you grow your own) and more expensive weight for weight, by consuming it you will be decreasing the number of chemicals you consume and thus increasing your nutrient intake. According to the Soil Association, organic vegetable foods are more nutrient-dense for the equivalent weight. As they have not been tampered with chemically they deliver much more of what nature promised.

The same is true for meat. Additive-free or organic meat has not been subjected to drugs, growth promoters or contaminated foods. This type of meat is now far more widely available than before (even our local high-street butcher supplies it, and some local farms and many supermarkets keep stocks). If you find 'clean' meat, it can be included in your diet approximately three times per week, unless of course you are vegetarian. An alternative is to limit your intake to lean meat, eat more fish, or become a vegetarian.

Often we have little control over environmental chemicals to which we are exposed, except to actively support a worthwhile campaign. However, there are other chemicals with which we have regular contact, that we can take or leave. You can do your bit for your health and the environment by implementing the following suggestions:

- Use ecologically safe cleaning agents at home
- Avoid using aerosols
- Use lead-free petrol
- Avoid using any chemicals if you're a keen gardener or grow vege-tables
- Do not use copper or aluminium saucepans
- Only use the microwave for reheating or defrosting
- Use filtered or bottled drinking water
- Avoid sitting for too long in front of a VDU on a regular basis
- Keep away from busy main roads – if you live on one try to move
- Do not spray pets with chemicals to prevent fleas
- Avoid paint that contains lead and do not sleep in a freshly painted room.

By eating a wholesome diet, rich in phytoestrogens, taking regular exercise and relaxation, and avoiding chemicals where possible, you can feel confident that you are actively working to maintain your health and increase your lifespan. In Part Two, Eating for Health, you will find exactly how to go about getting the best out of science on a day-by-day basis.

PART TWO

EATING FOR HEALTH – THE PHYTO FACTOR DIET

15

THE PRINCIPLES OF A PHYTOESTROGEN-RICH DIET

Consuming a diet rich in plant foods will provide dozens of different types of phytochemicals that possess health-protective benefits. Apart from soya products and linseeds which are rich sources of phytoestrogens, nuts, whole grains, fruits and vegetables contain an abundance of phenolic compounds, terpenoids, pigments and other natural antioxidants that have been associated with protection from, and in some cases treatment of, chronic diseases such as heart disease, cancer, diabetes, hypertension and a whole host of other medical conditions. Before launching into rules and recommendation of a diet that incorporates all these and more, let me assure you that the plan you are about to embark upon is both nutritious and enjoyable. It is not necessarily a vegetarian diet, unless you desire it to be so. Instead it is a simple regime that will supply all the nutrients you need, including what science currently dictates is the optimum amount of phytoestrogens to achieve the following:

- Dramatically reduce your risk of heart disease
- Keep your cholesterol levels within the normal range
- Help to keep your blood glucose levels on an even keel
- Reduce symptoms of the menopause and allow you to raise your oestrogen levels naturally each day
- Help to maintain your bone mass, reducing the risk of osteoporosis

ENJOYABLE EATING

Eating should be satisfying and fun. Meals need not be complex, intricate affairs in order to be nutritious, but can be simple and quick to prepare. The Women's Nutritional Advisory Service has provided specialised dietary advice to tens of thousands of people over the last 17 years, and as a result of the vast experience we have enjoyed as a team, we have managed to formulate recommendations that, as well as being enjoyable, are:

- Easy to prepare, including nutritious fast options for those who have limited time to spend in the kitchen
- Composed of a wide variety of fresh ingredients that are readily available in supermarkets and healthfood shops
- Suitable for the whole family
- Well balanced, providing a complete range of nutrients
- Wholesome snacks that maintain blood sugar levels and, additionally, provide a daily booster of plant oestrogens.

As you will come to realise, a truly healthy diet does not need to be faddy or complicated, nor does it require you to eat boring food or to count calories. Instead, you can simply enjoy the delights of eating tasty food, at the same time as reaping the health benefits. A further bonus of consuming predominantly wholesome fresh, plant-based foods instead of pre-prepared, refined foods, is that you are unlikely to add to the cost of your food bill; however, you are quite likely to add to the length of your life!

The recommendations have been designed to provide a healthy diet with a good balance of all the important nutrients. The portion sizes, where suggested, are average and should be adjusted according to your appetite, weight and activity level.

A word about soya

Soya products have traditionally received a bad press in the Western world. This is confirmed by the faces that many of our patients pull when we first suggest that they include soya products in their diet as one of the richest sources of phytoestrogens.

I have to confess, before going any further, that when I set out to write about including soya products in the diet on a regular basis, I was not personally a fan of soya products. Working with patients over the years, with the aim of persuading them to make dietary changes, has led me to be somewhat sneaky. I realised that it would be difficult for many people to eat and enjoy tofu kebabs for example. So I set out to disguise soya within the recipes for the reluctant vegetarians. To convince you of my success, let me relate an after-dinner story. Whilst preparing the sweet recipes for the book, we were having a dinner party. That evening I planned to serve three dessert options, and I decided to serve the Prune and Tofu Dessert, which you will find on page 228. I did cheat a little with the disguise, by serving it in individual chocolate cases, with a stoned prune on the top and chocolate shavings. To my surprise and utter delight, two of the women at the dinner asked for the recipe, and barely believed me when I told them it was made from fruit and tofu! This was a milestone, and I realised that I had cracked the problem.

From then on it has been easy and enjoyable for patients to incorporate tofu and soya products into their diets on a regular basis, without making major changes to their usual diets or spending hours on end in the kitchen. We developed a recipe for a phytoestrogen-rich muesli that we suggest serving with So Good soya milk, which is made from protein isolate, and has a good flavour. We also developed a number of fruit and tofu whips, which are very acceptable desserts or high-protein snacks, and a selection of fruit shakes, made in seconds in the blender with the fruit of your choice and So Good. There are also many recipes for bread, fruit loaves, cakes and biscuits, which will appeal to those who enjoy baking. For those who prefer savoury foods there are also a number of delicious dips which can be devoured with fresh vegetable *crudités* and corn chips.

Recent research regarding the frequency of phytoestrogen intake has confirmed our observations with our own patients. As phytoestrogens reach their peak in our bloodstream within approximately six to eight hours, it is important to consume phytoestrogens little and often. Ideally, you should start the day with a phytoestrogen-rich breakfast, have at least one other 'phyto fix' later in the day, and preferably a further serving, like a fruit shake or a slice of phyto fruit loaf in the evening, unless you choose to consume a vegetarian meal containing soya protein.

Another factor to bear in mind is that antibiotics interfere with the absorption of phytoestrogens, during the course of treatment and for at least six weeks, and possibly three months, after the course has terminated. If you have taken antibiotics recently you should be taking a probiotic containing lactobacilus acidophilus, whilst consuming your phytoestrogens, for at least three months, in order to restore the beneficial bacterial flora in your gut. If you do take antibiotics whilst you are following the WNAS menopause programme, you may experience a resurgence of your menopause symptoms. It is probably wise to avoid taking antibiotics for minor complaints whilst experiencing menopausal symptoms, and perhaps to use the herb, echinacea, to boost your immune system, or homeopathic remedies.

INGREDIENTS FOR A HEALTHY DIET

(Vegetarian options follow)

Meat and poultry   Always use lean cuts and trim the excess fat. Consume a maximum of three servings of red meat per week; preferably use poultry and game.

Fish   Consume at least three portions of oily fish per week, preferably fresh mackerel, herring, salmon, pilchards or sardines, which are all rich in the omega-3 series of essential fatty acids. Other fish and shellfish may be included in your diet.

Legumes   Include a variety of beans in your diet, preferably daily, but at least three or four times per week. Varieties include mung beans, which are a rich source of phytoestrogen, chick peas, lentils, kidney beans, split peas, black-eyed beans, aduki beans, lima beans and baked beans.

Soya products   Chapter 5 discussed the benefits of soya products, but we now need to look at just how much soya one needs to consume to get the maximum amount of benefit. The research currently indicates that as well as soya milk and yogurt, which contain relatively low levels of isoflavones, we should aim to consume at least one serving of soya protein per day. A serving is the equivalent of half a mug of tofu, tempeh, textured vegetarian protein or soya beans. Tofu, tempeh, soya beans, soya protein isolate and soya flour have a much higher content of isoflavones than soya milk, yogurt and ice cream. Refer to the chart on page 66.

Soya milk and yogurt   Aim to use soya milk and soya yogurt, which are available from both supermarkets and healthfood shops. Different brands of both soya milk and yogurt do vary in flavour, so you may need to experiment until you find the brands you prefer. Many of our patients have found the flavour of So Good soya drinks more acceptable than other brands. It is made from soya protein isolate, which means it does not have the beany flavour that seems to have put people off soya milk. A 250-ml glass of So Good will deliver approximately 25 mg of isoflavones. You can pour it on your Phyto Muesli at breakfast time, and use it in soups and baking, as heat does not interfere with the isoflavone content. In addition, unlike some other brands of soya milk, So Good can be used in piping hot tea, coffee and their substitutes, and it makes an excellent base for fruit shakes. So Good is a well-known Australian brand that has existed for over a hundred years. The first of the products in the range, So Good soya milk, was introduced to the United Kingdom just over a year ago. It is fortified with vitamins and minerals, in particular calcium, which means that it delivers as much calcium as cows' milk. As well as the regular flavour, it is now available as So Good Lite, a low-fat variety, and several fruit flavours including vanilla, strawberry and chocolate. It is widely available from all supermarkets.

Dairy milk and yogurt   Where possible use organic milk, preferably semi-skimmed, which is now available from supermarkets. Try to consume live yogurt (bio yogurt) because it restores a healthy gut flora. Aim to consume between half and one pint of milk per day. If you are not keen on dairy milk, use soya milk and yogurt instead, and concentrate on eating plenty of other calcium-rich foods (see page 289).

Cheese   A variety of cheeses is permitted, but bear in mind that cheese is a rich source of animal fat.

Eggs   Preferably free-range eggs may be consumed daily if desired, with a maximum of seven eggs per week.

Nuts and seeds   A variety of nuts and seeds should be included in your diet. Approximately two tablespoons of organic linseeds should be consumed daily, provided they sit happily in your gut. It is sometimes necessary to sprinkle one tablespoon on your breakfast cereal, and use the other serving over fruit after your dinner in the evening. Other seeds, including sunflower, sesame and pumpkin, also contain phytostrogens and can be eaten as a snack, included in cooking, or sprinkled on salads. Eat a variety of unsalted nuts, including almonds, pecans, walnuts, pine nuts, pistachios, cashews and peanuts. Nut butters, including peanut, almond or mixed nut can be spread on bread or used in dips, as can tahini, which is sesame seed butter.

Fruit, vegetables and salad   People who eat greater amounts of fruits, vegetables and salad have about half the risk of becoming cancer victims and much less chance of dying from cancer than those who eat less. The Five a Day campaigns that have been running in both the UK and the USA are designed to heighten awareness about the health properties of fruit and vegetables. However, a survey conducted in the USA confirmed that only one person in eleven was meeting the guidelines for fruit and vegetables. One in every nine surveyed ate no fruit or vegetables at all, and a massive 45 per cent ate no fruit on the day of the survey. Citrus fruits, including oranges, grapefruits and lemons, in addition to providing an ample supply of vitamin C, folic acid, potassium and pectin, contain a host of active phytochemicals that can protect our health. More than 60 flavonoids found in citrus fruit have been found to have anti-inflammatory properties, anti-tumour activity, strong anti-oxidant activity and to inhibit the formation of blood clots. Oranges alone contain more than 170 phytochemicals. Therefore, aim to eat three portions of fresh fruit per day (one bowl of berries, or an apple or orange = one portion). Fresh fruit is preferable, although tinned fruit in natural juice is permitted. Vegetables have also been shown to have anti-cancer properties, and many contain phytoestrogens (see list on page 55). Three portions of fresh vegetables should be consumed daily, including one green leafy vegetable, e.g. cabbage, spinach, broccoli, kale, Brussels sprouts, cauliflower, and one yellow vegetable, e.g. carrots, tomatoes or peppers. Additionally, garlic and onions, which are members of the sulphide-rich allium family, seem to play a significant part in protecting us from both cancer and heart disease. Where possible have raw vegetables in salads and raw vegetable *crudités*. Cook vegetables in the minimum amount of water, or steam if possible to preserve the nutrients. In addition to this, you should ideally include a daily salad in your diet.

Whole grains   The phytochemicals found in fruit and vegetables are very similar to those in whole grains, and include plant sterols. These substances have been found to reduce the risk of cardiovascular disease and cancer. Try to incorporate a variety of grains into your diet as well as wheat, including rye, oats, corn and rice. Healthfood shops often stock a good variety of breads made from alternative flours to wheat.

Fried food   Use the stir-fry method with a minimum of oil and keep other fried foods to a minimum.

Oils and fats   Use polyunsaturated oils, e.g. sunflower, rape, walnut and sesame, soya and linseed. Polyunsaturated spreads like Flora are preferable to butter. Small amounts of butter can be used on toast or crackers if preferred.

Sugar and sweet foods   Keep sugar-rich foods to a minimum and always consume them after a wholesome meal. Refined sugar does not contain any vitamins or minerals whatsoever, but does demand good nutrients in order to be metabolised. Options for cooking include fructose (fruit sugars), concentrated apple juice and small amounts of honey.

Salt and salty foods   Try not to add salt to cooking or at the table especially if fluid retention is a problem, or if you suffer with high blood pressure, as salt tends to drag fluid into the cells. We already consume far too much salt. If you enjoy the salty flavour, use LoSalt or a similar potassium-rich substitute.

Tea and coffee   Avoid caffeine and keep decaffeinated teas and coffees to a maximum of four cups per day. Ideally try some of the alternatives listed on page 159–60.

Herbs   A number of herbs, including rosemary, sage, oregano and thyme, belong to the *Labiatae* family and are known to possess strong anti-oxidant properties. Ginger contains a dozen phenolic compounds, known as gingerols, which have even greater anti-oxidant activity than vitamin E.

DIETARY RULES

- Eat three proper meals a day
- Always start the day with breakfast – it is the most important meal of the day
- Plan your meals ahead, preferably a week in advance so that when you go shopping you can make sure you purchase the correct ingredients
- Eat wholesome snacks between meals to keep your blood sugar constant particularly in your premenstrual week if you are menstruating
- Avoid convenience foods and junk food, which is high in sugar, salt or fat
- Go shopping at least twice a week to buy fresh fruit and vegetables
- Don't go shopping on an empty stomach as you may end up buying the wrong foods. Take a list with you and try to stick to it
- Arrange to eat with family and friends as often as possible
- Savour your food as you eat and chew it well.

Alternatives to caffeine

It is particularly important for people suffering with nervous tension, mood swings, irritability, headaches, breast tenderness or insomnia to avoid caffeine. Many alternatives are listed below, but beware the withdrawal symptoms. Often in the first week of avoiding caffeine people experience extra symptoms of headaches, anxiety, irritability, mood swings, insomnia and sometimes fatigue. These symptoms do pass within the space of a few days to a week, so do persist.

Follow the basic dietary recommendations, but avoid caffeine in the form of tea, coffee, chocolate, chocolate drinks and cola-based drinks. Read labels carefully as often painkillers contain caffeine.

Look out for alternative products which are available from the supermarkets and healthfood shops.

Herbal teas　Fruit teas like raspberry and ginseng, fennel, and ginseng tea all contain a small amount of naturally occurring oestrogen. Other favourites include lemon verbena, lemon and ginger with a slice of lemon, and the mixed berry varieties. There is a wide variety of choices available and very often they are sold in single sachets so that you can buy and try without being committed to a whole box of tea bags.

Rooisbosch, Red Bush or Rooi Tea   A very tea-like alternative to tea when made with milk, but contains no caffeine, very little tannin and a mild muscle relaxant. There are a number of other teas available in healthfood shops that fit into this category.

Coffee   There are a variety of substitutes for coffee, including Barley Cup, Carro, Bambu and No Caf, which are all worth trying. In addition Teeccino is a wonderful new filter coffee supplement which comes in a variety of flavours. Dandelion coffee is also pleasant and it comes in two varieties; the instant, which comes in a jar and is sweet and the dandelion root, which can be purchased in a healthfood shop, ground in a coffee grinder and stored in a jar. This is best used through a coffee filter or strainer, either over a cup or through a coffee filter machine. It makes a very strong malted drink.

Fizzy drinks   There are many sparkling drinks available to take the place of cola-based drinks and other fizzy drinks that contain caffeine. Most supermarkets sell their own brand as well as leading makes like Appletise, Irish Spring, Ami, Aqua Libra, etc.

Chocolate   If you are avoiding caffeine completely, chocolate will have to go too. There are a few non-dairy alternatives that are perfectly acceptable, which usually contain carob and soya. The alternatives can usually be found in healthfood shops. Eating fresh fruit or dried fruits, nuts and seeds, which are intrinsically sweet foods on which our ancestors relied, is in any case a much more nutritious alternative to snacking on chocolate.

16

VEGETARIAN OR VEGAN OPTIONS

A vegetarian should strictly mean someone who eats only vegetable derived foods, but a strict vegetarian is now more usually referred to as a vegan. 'Vegetarian' is often used to describe somebody who simply avoids meat, fish and poultry, but this can be further subdivided. Those who consume dairy products as well are known as lacto-vegetarian, and those who consume eggs as well as dairy products are known as ovo-lacto-vegetarian.

According to the Realeat Survey conducted by the Gallup Organisation in 1997, over the previous two years in the UK alone, 5,000 individuals became vegetarians, which is an increase of over 20 per cent when compared with a previous 1995 survey. In addition to this over 13,000 people every week for the previous two years had stopped eating red meat, and almost half the population are now actively eating less red meat. Obviously BSE has been cited as the prime motivation for people to make this major lifestyle change. Vegetarians can consume a perfectly nutritious diet, but they have to work harder to ensure that they consume a full complement of nutrients than their meat-eating counterparts.

INGREDIENTS FOR A HEALTHY VEGETARIAN DIET

- Avoid refined carbohydrates as they are low in essential minerals and vitamins. It is advisable that they should only be consumed in very small quantities by vegetarians and vegans. The intake of essential nutrients, particularly iron and zinc, may be borderline in some vegetarians and vegans and this will only be further hindered by consuming refined carbohydrates.
- Ensure an adequate balance of protein in your diet. A major problem with vegetarian and vegan diets has been borderline, or poor quality protein intake. This is particularly true in those who have not taken care to learn the protein-rich foods or their combinations that vegetarians and vegans should eat. Protein-rich foods include

nuts, seeds, peas, beans, lentils, whole grains, brown rice, sprouted beans and soya bean preparations. Vegetarians and vegans should not rely heavily upon any one source of vegetable protein.

If you are not a strict vegan, make use of other protein-rich foods. High-quality, well-balanced protein is found in eggs, which are also rich in iron. One or two eggs can be consumed quite safely per day and would be beneficial.

Protein combination

- Rice with legumes, chick peas, lentils, sesame or cheese
- Wheat with legumes or mixed nuts and milk or sesame and soya beans
- Corn with legumes
- Mixed nuts with sunflower seeds
- Sesame seeds with beans **or** mixed nuts and soya beans **or** mixed nuts and soya beans **or** wheat and soya beans

The addition of any first-class protein, e.g. milk, or particularly eggs may substantially enhance the protein value of the vegetable food. Not all members of the legume family are high in protein. Those that are particularly nutritious include:

• mung beans	• lentils
• red kidney beans	• peas
• haricot beans	• split peas
• butter beans	• soya beans
• chick peas	

Sprouted beans may be more appetising. Soaking beans for 24 hours and de-husking them may reduce the problem of wind, which occurs in some bean eaters.

Avoid foods that block mineral absorption

Many foods contain substances that bind with essential trace minerals and prevent their absorption. Such foods include bran, unleavened wheat – particularly wholewheat as in pastry or when used as a thickening agent – tea, coffee, soft drinks and foods containing phosphate additives. Alcohol also causes increased losses of trace minerals. Iron and zinc absorption may be inhibited by the above foods and drinks, which should be avoided or consumed in small quantities. It should never be necessary for a vegetarian or vegan to eat bran as there is plenty of fibre in other foods. Also tea should not be consumed with vegetarian meals because of its powerful effect in reducing iron absorption. It is suggested, therefore, that tea consumption should be minimal, two or fewer cups per day, particularly in female vegetarians.

Ensure an adequate supply of mineral- and vitamin-rich foods. Usually, if you are careful to balance the quantities of protein in your diet and avoid mineral-depleted convenience foods, your intake of trace minerals should, on the whole, be good. It is strongly recommended that vegetarians and vegans learn which foods are nutritious. The worst possible combination is a poor quality vegetarian diet and a high intake of sweets, chocolates and other nutrient-depleted foods.

VEGETARIAN AND VEGANS IN SPECIAL SITUATIONS

There are certain situations when a vegetarian or vegan diet may be distinctly inadvisable, or should only be undertaken if one has a very good knowledge of what a healthy vegetarian diet is. Those particularly at risk include:

- infants under the age of one year as well as young children
- the elderly, pregnant or breastfeeding women
- people who are ill or who have nutritional deficiencies.

Usually medical advice should be sought, in particular to determine whether any additional supplements may be required by people in such situations. Infants, for example, may frequently become short of iron on a strict vegetarian or vegan diet. Severe vegan diets may, in fact, lead to rickets in young children because of lack of vitamin D and calcium in the diet.

The nutritional requirements of pregnant and breastfeeding women must be met and a poor quality vegetarian diet will often not be sufficient. Specific advice about the use of supplements in the pre-conceptual phase, during pregnancy and when breastfeeding can be found in *Healthy Parents, Healthy Baby* (see page 257 for details).

The elderly have a declining food intake and so the quality of their dietary intake must be very high in order for them not to develop deficiencies.

While there are certain medical conditions that would be benefited by undertaking a vegetarian or vegan diet, patients who are ill or who have nutritional deficiencies should seek medical advice before embarking on such a programme.

FOOD ALLERGY AND VEGETARIANS

Food allergies are increasingly common and the major foods that appear to cause trouble are wheat, milk, yeast and sometimes even soya products, many of which may be staple foods in a vegetarian or vegan diet. Thus, if after embarking upon a vegetarian or vegan diet your health deteriorates, it may be because of inadequacies in the diet or the presence of food allergies or intolerances. On the other hand certain aspects of vegetarian or vegan diets may be beneficial for people with food allergies or intolerances, in particular the high consumption of salads and vegetables. If you suspect you may have food allergies you may need to seek advice, or follow one of the exclusion diets in the book *Every Woman's Health Guide* or the plan in my new *Zest for Life Plan* (for details see page 257).

Vitamin B12

Many experienced vegetarians and vegans appreciate the importance of ensuring adequate vitamin B12 in the diet. The major source of vitamin B12 is meat. Other reasonably good sources include eggs, brewer's yeast and dairy produce, and tempeh, the soya bean patty. Only strict vegans may need a vitamin B12 supplement. However, anyone who develops vitamin B12 deficiency should receive appropriate investigations to determine precisely the cause of their deficiency; it should not be presumed to be due to dietary inadequacy, but may be due to absorbency problems.

For suggested vegetarian menus, please go to Chapter 18, pages 174–78.

17

THE FOUR-WEEK MENU PLAN

A SAMPLE MENU SELECTION FOR FOUR WEEKS

Recipes marked with an asterisk and fast-option menus can be found in Chapter 19.

WEEK ONE

Day 1

BREAKFAST
Porridge made with So Good
   soya milk
Almonds
Sunflower seeds, pumpkin seeds
Banana, chopped

LUNCH
Scrambled tofu*
Rye bread, toasted
Pilchards

DINNER
Chicken with almond sauce*
Green beans
Sweetcorn
Jacket potato

DESSERT
Prune and tofu whip*

SNACKS
Dried apricots
Almond biscuit*

Day 2

BREAKFAST
Soya yogurt
Apple, chopped
Sunflower seeds, pumpkin seeds
Pecan nuts, chopped

LUNCH
Cauliflower soup*
Oatcakes or French bread
1 apple

DINNER
Soya bean casserole*
New potatoes
Peas
Carrots

DESSERT
Cinnamon rhubarb* with soya
   yogurt

SNACKS
Orange
Honey soya loaf *

Day 3

BREAKFAST
Crunchy almond muesli* with So
    Good soya milk
Pear, chopped

LUNCH
Jacket potato
Refried soya beans*
Green salad
Apple

DINNER
Baked chicken burgers with
    almond chilli dressing*
Rice
Sweetcorn
Broccoli

DESSERT
Apple and cinnamon crumble*
    with soya custard

SNACKS
Banana
Mixed unsalted nuts

Day 4

BREAKFAST
Banana oat pancakes* with soya
    yogurt and chopped fresh fruit

LUNCH
Sesame tofu* with tahini
    mayonnaise*
Tropical rice salad*
Apple

DINNER
Polenta pie*
Rice
Roasted vegetables

DESSERT
Blackberry and rhubarb
    compote*
Soya Dream or soya yogurt

SNACKS
Pear
Rice cakes with nut butter
Sunflower seeds, pumpkin
    seeds

Day 5

BREAKFAST
Rice porridge* made with So
    Good soya milk
Dried apricots
Almonds
Sesame seeds

LUNCH
Watercress soup*
Soya and cornbread*
Small piece of cheese
Apple

DINNER
Shepherdess pie*
Cauliflower
Carrots

DESSERT
Tofu orange almond dessert*

SNACKS
Oatcakes with pure fruit
    spread
Banana

Day 6

BREAKFAST
Soya and raisin loaf*
Banana smoothie* with Phyto
   sprinkle*

LUNCH
Jacket potato with spicy soya
   beans*
Coleslaw*

DINNER
Baked avocado with tuna*
Endive, fruit and nut salad*
New potatoes

DESSERT
Banana and tofu cream*

SNACKS
Sesame squares*
Peach whiz*

Day 7

BREAKFAST
Crunchy almond muesli* with So
   Good soya milk
Pear, chopped

LUNCH
Burgen bread
Soya cheese
Apple and nut salad*

DINNER
Salmon potato cakes* with
   avocado sauce*
Tropical rice salad*

DESSERT
Ginger fruit salad*
Soya Dream

SNACKS
Cinnamon flapjack*
Banana and date shake*

WEEK TWO

Day 1

BREAKFAST
Phyto muesli* with So Good
   soya milk
Pear, chopped

LUNCH
Tempeh kebab with pitta bread*
Apple

DINNER
Prawn and almond risotto*
Green beans
Sweetcorn

DESSERT
Rhubarb fool with tofu lemon
   sauce*

SNACKS
Dried apricots
Chocolate fruit slice*

Day 2

BREAKFAST
Cornflakes with So Good soya
   milk
Raisins
Pecan nuts
Sunflower seeds, pumpkin seeds

LUNCH
Bean tacos* with green salad
Apple

DINNER
Salmon steaks with orange and
    ginger sauce*
New potatoes
Courgettes
Carrots

DESSERT
Fruit and nut compote*
Soya yogurt

SNACKS
Buckwheat scone* with pure
    fruit spread
Pear

Day 3

BREAKFAST
Puffed rice cereal with So Good
    soya milk
Banana, chopped
Pecan nuts, chopped
Phyto sprinkle*

LUNCH
Herbed tofu pâté*
Oatcakes
Rice salad with pumpkin seeds,
    sunflower seeds and nuts

DINNER
Yogurt roast chicken*
Swede
Roast potatoes
Carrots
Cabbage

DESSERT
Baked banana and rice
    pudding*

SNACKS
Ginger snaps*
Apple

Day 4

BREAKFAST
Porridge made with So Good
    soya milk
Almonds
Dried apricots
Phyto sprinkle*

LUNCH
Scrambled tofu*
Oatcakes and soya cheese
Apple

DINNER
Lamb stir-fry with almonds and
    walnuts*
Rice noodles

DESSERT
Banana lemon whip*

SNACKS
Barley scone* with pure fruit spread
Banana

Day 5

BREAKFAST
Cornflakes with So Good soya milk
Banana, chopped
Almonds
Phyto sprinkle*

LUNCH
Carrot soup*
Soya and cornbread*
Soya cheese

DINNER
Nutty tofu risotto*
Orange and avocado salad*

DESSERT
Tofu strawberry dessert*

SNACKS
Chewy fruit bar*
Pear

Day 6

BREAKFAST
Scrambled tofu*
Grilled tomato and mushrooms
Grilled tempeh
Slice toast

LUNCH
Jacket potato with barbecued
    soya beans*
Green salad
Apple

DINNER
Prawn and spinach curry*
Rice
Poppadum

DESSERT
Apricot squares* with soya custard
    (made from So Good soya milk)

SNACKS
Honey loaf*, toasted
Mixed nuts

Day 7

BREAKFAST
Soya yogurt
Fresh fruit of your choice
Almonds and pecan nuts
Phyto sprinkle*

LUNCH
Mushroom omelette
Green salad
Pear

DINNER
Stuffed pepper*
Rice
Green beans
Sweetcorn

DESSERT
Apple and tofu cheesecake*

SNACKS
Apricot coconut balls*
Banana

WEEK THREE

Day 1

BREAKFAST
Rice porridge* made with So
    Good soya milk
Dried apricots
Almonds, chopped

LUNCH
Soya and buckwheat pancakes*
    with refried soya beans*
Green salad
Pear

DINNER
Lamb kebabs with mint yogurt
    sauce*
Rice
Sweetcorn
Green beans

DESSERT
Rhubarb and ginger mousse*

SNACKS
Fruit smoothie*
Oatcakes with nut butter

Day 2

BREAKFAST
Phyto muesli* with So Good
    soya milk
Banana, chopped

LUNCH
Jacket potato with spicy soya beans*
Endive, fruit and nut salad*

DINNER
Grilled tuna steak with orange
    sauce*
New potatoes
Carrots
Broccoli

DESSERT
Chocolate pie with passion
    fruit sauce*

SNACKS
Seed bread*, toasted with pure
    fruit spread
Dried apricots

Day 3

BREAKFAST
Cornflakes with So Good soya milk
Banana, chopped
Almonds
Phyto sprinkle*

LUNCH
Tofu tuna spread*
Rye bread
Green salad

DINNER
Lentil dahl*
Basmati rice
Poppadum

DESSERT
Ginger fruit salad*
Soya Dream or soya yogurt

SNACKS
Rice, soya and raisin bread* with
    pure fruit spread
Apple
Sunflower seeds and pumpkin
    seeds

Day 4

BREAKFAST
Scrambled tofu*
Grilled mushrooms
Rye bread, toasted

LUNCH
Leek, sweetcorn and almond soup*
Rye bread toasted
Pear

DINNER
Italian corn pasta*
Sweetcorn
Broccoli

DESSERT
Rhubarb crumble*
Soya Dream or soya custard (made
    with So Good soya milk)

SNACKS
Banana smoothie*
Barley scone*

Day 5

BREAKFAST
Crunchy almond muesli* with
    with soya yogurt
Banana, chopped

LUNCH
Hummus* and raw vegetables
Oatcakes
Apple

DINNER
Spicy chilli*
Green salad
Sweetcorn

DESSERT
Elderflower sorbet*

SNACKS
Rhubarb and blackberry smoothie*
Apple

Day 6

BREAKFAST
Phyto muesli* with So Good
   soya milk
Banana, chopped

LUNCH
Pilchards
Oatcakes
Carrot and raisin salad*
Apple

DINNER
Tofu 'meat' balls*
Rice
Sweet potato salad*

DESSERT
Stewed apple and rhubarb
Soya yogurt or soya custard

SNACKS
Nutty flapjack*
Pear

Day 7

BREAKFAST
Banana oat pancakes* with soya
   yogurt and honey

LUNCH
Potato skins with broccoli and
   tofu filling*
Green salad
Apple

DINNER
Prawn kebabs with peanut chilli
   sauce*
Rice
Sweetcorn
Green salad

DESSERT
Apricot squares*
Soya custard

SNACKS
Honey loaf*
Apple

WEEK FOUR

Day 1

BREAKFAST
Cornflakes with So Good soya
   milk
Dried apricots
Almonds

LUNCH
Cauliflower soup*
Rye bread
Apple

DINNER
Lentil bolognese*
Green salad

DESSERT
Banana and tofu cream*

SNACKS
Ginger snaps*
Mixed nuts

171

Day 2

BREAKFAST
Puffed rice cereal with So Good
    soya milk
Banana, chopped
Pecans, chopped

LUNCH
Carrot and apricot pâté*
Oatcakes
Green salad
Pear

DINNER
'Lasagne'*
Roasted vegetables
Green salad

DESSERT
Fruit and nut compote*
Soya Dream or soya yogurt

SNACKS
Honey loaf*
Pear

Day 3

BREAKFAST
Phyto muesli* with So Good
    soya milk
Banana, chopped

LUNCH
Hummus* with *crudités*
Rice cakes
Apple

DINNER
Chicken kebabs* with tamari
    and ginger dressing*
Jacket potato
Brown rice and watercress salad*

DESSERT
Apple and tofu cheesecake*
Soya Dream

SNACKS
Parkin*
Mixed unsalted nuts

Day 4

BREAKFAST
Breakfast rice cakes* with soya
    yogurt and pure fruit spread
Banana

LUNCH
Sesame tofu*
Green salad

DINNER
Lamb steaks with pomegranate
    and walnut sauce*
Green beans
Broccoli
Carrots

DESSERT
Baked rice and banana pudding*
Dried apricots, chopped

SNACKS
Buckwheat scone*
Soya yogurt with chopped dried
    apricots and mixed nuts

Day 5

BREAKFAST
Porridge made with So Good
    soya milk
Dried apricots
Almonds

LUNCH
Jacket potato with barbecued
    soya beans*
Green salad
Banana

DINNER
Chicken and almond pilaff*
Sweetcorn
Green beans

DESSERT
Chocolate and fruit slice*

SNACKS
Honey loaf*, toasted
Apple

Day 6

BREAKFAST
Phyto muesli* with So Good
    soya milk
Banana, chopped

LUNCH
Rye bread sandwich with tofu
    tuna spread*
Apple and nut salad*

DINNER
Soya bean biryani*
Vegetable curry
Poppadum

DESSERT
Ginger fruit salad* with Soya
    Dream

SNACKS
Almond loaf*
Banana

Day 7

BREAKFAST
Soya yogurt
Kiwi fruit, banana, chopped
Almonds, pumpkin seeds
Dried apricots

LUNCH
Refried soya beans* with jacket
    potato
Green salad

DINNER
Cod with orange and almonds*
New potatoes
Green beans
Carrots

DESSERT
Prune and tofu dessert*

SNACKS
Sesame square*
Pear

18

THE VEGETARIAN PLAN

VEGETARIAN SAMPLE MENUS FOR TWO WEEKS

Recipes marked with an asterisk can be found in Chapter 19.

WEEK ONE

Day 1

BREAKFAST
Scrambled tofu*
Grilled tomatoes and
    mushrooms
Rye bread, toasted

LUNCH
Cauliflower soup*
Oatcakes
Apple

DINNER
Tofu, bean and herb stir-fry*
Rice

DESSERT
Fruit and nut compote*
Soya Dream

SNACKS
Apricot and coconut balls*
Pear

Day 2

BREAKFAST
Rice porridge*
Raisins, dried apricots

LUNCH
Hummus*
Soya and cornbread*
Apple

DINNER
Spinach gratin*
Jacket potato
Carrots
Sweetcorn

DESSERT
Stewed apple and blackberries
    with soya custard (made with
    So Good soya milk)*

SNACKS
Apple bread roll* with pure
    fruit spread
Almonds

Day 3

BREAKFAST
Dried fruit compote*
Almonds
Soya yogurt

LUNCH
Savoury crackers*
Soya cheese
Orange and avocado salad*

DINNER
Hungarian bean goulash*
Sauté potatoes
Cauliflower
Carrots

DESSERT
Rhubarb fool with tofu lemon
    cream*

SNACKS
Almond and cinnamon
    flapjack*
Banana

Day 4

BREAKFAST
Cornflakes and puffed rice cereal
    with So Good soya milk
Almonds, pecan nuts
Dried apricots

LUNCH
Carrot and almond pâté*
Oatcakes
Green salad

DINNER
Leek gratin*
New potatoes
Carrots
Courgettes

DESSERT
Chocolate tofu berry whip*

SNACKS
Sesame slice*
Apple

Day 5

BREAKFAST
Poached egg
Rye bread, toasted
Banana

LUNCH
Avocado, smoked tofu and
    pineapple salad*
Apple bun*

DINNER
Indonesian tofu kebabs with
    satay sauce*
Stir-fried mixed vegetables
Rice noodles

DESSERT
Tofu cheesecake*

SNACKS
Dried apricots
Almonds

Day 6

BREAKFAST
Soya yogurt
Banana and pear, chopped
Oatcakes and marmalade

LUNCH
Bean tacos*
Orange and avocado salad*

DINNER
Broccoli and smoked tofu*
New potatoes
Carrots
Sweetcorn

DESSERT
Nut crunch with tofu whipped
    cream*

SNACKS
Almond biscuit*
Pear
Mixed nuts

Day 7

BREAKFAST
Phyto muesli* with So Good
    soya milk
Pear, chopped

LUNCH
Jacket potato with hummus*
Green salad
Apple

DINNER
Carrot and nut loaf* with
    tahini and lemon dressing*
Sweet potato salad*
Courgettes

DESSERT
Rhubarb crumble* with soya
    custard

SNACKS
Fruit chewy bar*
Pear

WEEK TWO

Day 1

BREAKFAST
Rice porridge*
Banana, chopped
Almonds

LUNCH
Leek, sweetcorn and almond
    soup*
Rye bread, toasted
Apple

DINNER
Barley roast with tahini sauce*
New potatoes
Sweetcorn
Broccoli

DESSERT
Ginger and fruit salad*
Soya yogurt

SNACKS
Apricot and coconut balls*
Pear

Day 2

BREAKFAST
Porridge made with So Good
    soya milk*
Banana, chopped
Dried apricots

LUNCH
Jacket potato
Tuna in soya oil
Green salad
Apple

DINNER
Shepherdess pie*
Carrots
Cabbage

DESSERT
Tofu orange and almond dessert*

SNACKS
Sesame squares*
Pear

Day 3

BREAKFAST
Cornflakes with So Good soya milk
Almonds
Banana, chopped

LUNCH
Tempeh kebabs with pitta bread*
Apple

DINNER
Noodles in spicy sesame sauce*
Stir-fried mixed vegetables

DESSERT
Prune and tofu dessert*

SNACKS
Honey loaf*
Pear

Day 4

BREAKFAST
Banana oat pancakes* with soya
    yogurt
Apple

LUNCH
Carrot and apricot pâté*
Rye bread, toasted
Pear

DINNER
Red lentil dhal* with basmati rice
Poppadum

DESSERT
Banana raisin whip*

SNACKS
Oatcakes with pure fruit spread
Dried apricots
Mixed unsalted nuts

Day 5

BREAKFAST
Cornflakes with So Good soya milk
Dried apricots
Pumpkin seeds and pecan nuts

LUNCH
Scrambled tofu*
Rye bread, toasted
Endive, fruit and nut salad*
Apple

DINNER
Lentil bolognese*
Spaghetti

DESSERT
Cinnamon rhubarb whip*

SNACKS
Chocolate fruit slice*
Pear

Day 6

BREAKFAST
Breakfast rice cakes* with
   mashed banana
Nut butter

LUNCH
Watercress soup*
Rye bread
Orange and avocado salad*

DINNER
Sesame tofu* with tahini
   dressing*
Stir-fried mixed vegetables
Rice noodles

DESSERT
Raspberry and tofu brûlée*

SNACKS
Orange and ginger cake*
Apple

Day 7

BREAKFAST
Rice porridge*
Banana, chopped
Almonds

LUNCH
Carrot and apricot pâté*
Oatcakes
Green salad

DINNER
Bean and tofu casserole*
Jacket potato
Green beans
Carrots

DESSERT
Prune and tofu whip*

SNACKS
Nutty flapjack*
Banana

19

RECIPES – DELICIOUS AND NUTRITIOUS

LUNCHES – FAST OPTIONS

(Recipes marked with an asterisk are given in this chapter.)

Raw vegetables and dips, e.g. hummus*, taramasalata
Refried soya beans* with corn tacos
Jacket potato with spicy soya beans*
Jacket potato with barbecued soya beans*
Omelette with salad (see salad selection)
Spicy soya beans* on rye toast
Stir-fried tofu and mixed vegetables with rice
Soup (see soup selection) and rye bread/corn and soya bread
Rice salad with pumpkin seeds, sunflower seeds and nuts
Fruit and nut compote* with soya yogurt
Scrambled tofu* with rye bread or jacket potato
Soya and buckwheat pancakes* with refried soya beans*
Grilled tempeh with salad
Bean tacos* with salad
Tempeh kebab with pitta bread*
Sesame tofu* with salad
Rye bread with soya cheese and salad
Oatcakes with nut butter and salad

DINNERS – FAST OPTIONS

Tofu kebabs with satay sauce* with stir-fried vegetables and rice
Tofu risotto*
Prawn and tofu kebabs with rice and salad
Lamb kebabs* with vegetables and rice
Salmon steaks with orange ginger sauce* and vegetables
Fresh pilchards, grilled and served with salad and new potatoes
Refried beans* with rice, corn chips and avocado
Stir-fried tofu and vegetables with rice noodles

Tofu burgers* with salad and a jacket potato
Baked avocado with tuna* with salad and a jacket potato
Stuffed pepper* with salad
Grilled lamb chop with rosemary* served with vegetables and new
   potatoes
Chicken kebabs with tamari and ginger dressing*
Spinach gratin* with a jacket potato
Tofu, bean and herb stir-fry* with rice
Noodles in spicy sesame sauce*
Cauliflower cheese with a jacket potato
Bubble and squeak with mackerel
Sesame tofu* with salad and a jacket potato

BREAKFASTS

SOYA AND RICE PANCAKES

50 g (2 oz) rice flour
50 g (2 oz) soya flour
1 small egg

300 ml (1/2 pint) So Good soya
   milk
a little soya oil

1. Make a thin batter with the flours, egg and So Good.
2. Use kitchen paper to wipe a small non-stick frying pan with a little
   oil and heat until the oil is smoking.
3. Pour a generous 2 tablespoons of batter into the pan and swirl it
   around to cover the base. Cook for 60 seconds.
4. Flip it over and cook for a further few seconds. Set aside.
5. Repeat the procedure until you have used up all the batter.

SERVES 4

BANANA OAT PANCAKES

50 g (2 oz) porridge oats
50 g (2 oz) soya flour
50 g (2 oz) rice flour
1 tbsp potassium-rich baking powder

150 ml (1/4 pint) So Good
   soya milk
2 bananas, thinly sliced

1. In a bowl, combine the oats, flours and baking powder. Add the
   So Good and blend well with the flour and oat mixture until a thin
   batter is formed. Fold in the banana slices.

2. Pour sufficient batter mixture into a lightly oiled non-stick frying pan and cook until bubbles appear on the surface. Flip the pancake over and cook on the other side for about 1 minute.
3. Serve the pancakes warm with pure maple syrup, soya yogurt and chopped fresh fruit.

MAKES 12

RICE PORRIDGE

100 g (4 oz) brown rice flakes
600 ml (1 pint) boiling water
1/4 tsp ground cloves

1/4 tsp ground cinnamon
1 piece fresh fruit, e.g. banana,
    apple

1. Place the rice flakes in the boiling water and cook for about 15 minutes until the rice is soft.
2. Add the ground cloves and cinnamon and serve with a piece of fresh fruit.

SERVES 2

buckwheat pancakes

50 g (2 oz) buckwheat flour
50 g (2 oz) soya flour
2 tbsp golden linseeds

300 ml (1/2 pint) So Good soya milk
sunflower oil

1. Mix all the ingredients until well combined and set aside.
2. Heat 1 tbsp of sunflower oil in a large frying pan and pour in enough mixture to coat the base, tilting the pan until the batter runs evenly all over. Cook for about 2 minutes until browned on the underside.
3. Turn the pancake over and cook the other side.
4. Serve with sweet or savoury fillings.

Serving suggestions
scrambled eggs
grilled bacon
cottage cheese and pineapple
maple syrup and banana
banana and chopped almonds
yogurt and chopped fresh fruit
stewed apple with cinnamon and chopped nuts

SERVES 4

Cinnamon Porridge

300 ml (1/2 pint) So Good soya milk
225 g (8 oz) rolled oats
2 tbsp golden linseeds
50 g (2 oz) ground almonds

1 tsp ground cinnamon
2 tbsp golden linseeds
soya 'cream'
pure maple syrup

1. Place the So Good, oats, linseeds and cinnamon into a saucepan and bring to the boil. Reduce the heat and simmer for about 5 minutes, stirring occasionally until the oats are soft.
2. Stir in the ground almonds and serve with soya cream and maple syrup to sweeten.

SERVES 2

Nutty Rice Pancakes

50 g (2 oz) wild rice, rinsed
1 tsp salt
25 g (1 oz) butter, melted
4 eggs, separated
300 ml (1/2 pint) So Good
  soya milk

100 g (4 oz) blanched, toasted
  almonds, finely chopped
50 g (2 oz) rice flour
50 g (2 oz) cornflour
pinch of cream of tartar
sunflower oil and butter for cooking

1. Bring 250 ml (8fl oz) water to the boil in a medium saucepan. Add the wild rice; cover and simmer over a low heat for about 45–55 minutes, until the rice is tender and all the water has been absorbed. Add the salt and the melted butter.
2. Whisk the egg yolks until they are a pale colour, then mix into the rice. Stir in the So Good, chopped nuts and flours. In a separate bowl, beat the egg whites with a pinch of cream of tartar until stiff, but not dry. Fold into the batter.
3. To cook the pancakes, melt 15 g (^{1}/2 oz) butter with 1 tbsp sunflower oil in a heavy-based frying pan or griddle over a medium heat. When hot, add spoonfuls of the batter to the pan to form 6-cm (2^1/2-inch) pancakes. Cook for 2–3 minutes until the edges are golden brown and the pancakes have begun to set. Flip the pancakes to brown the other side, then remove. Repeat with the remaining batter.
4. Arrange the hot pancakes in a single layer in an ovenproof dish; keep warm in the oven until all the pancakes are cooked.
5. Serve warm with fruit, maple syrup and yogurt.

MAKES 36

PHYTO SPRINKLE

An excellent source of phytoestrogens which can be conveniently combined with your daily diet. Use in bread and cake recipes or to sprinkle over breakfast cereals, salads and desserts

1/2 mug almonds
1/2 mug sunflower seeds

1/2 mug pumpkin seeds
1/2 mug golden linseeds

1. Grind the ingredients together in a blender to a coarse consistency.
2. Store in a sealed container. Keep refrigerated to prevent seeds from going rancid.

CRUNCHY ALMOND MUESLI

450 g (1 lb) rolled oats
100 g (4 oz) sunflower seeds
225 g (8 oz) chopped almonds
150 ml (1/4 pint) brown rice syrup
150 ml (1/4 pint) soya oil

150 ml (1/4 pint) unsweetened apple juice
225 g (8 oz) organic raisins
100 g (4 oz) desiccated coconut

1 Pre-heat the oven to 150°C/300°F/gas mark 2. Mix the oats, sunflower seeds and almonds together in a large bowl.
2. Blend the syrup, oil and apple juice in a jug and pour over the oat and almond mixture.
3. Spread this mixture on to a baking tray and bake for 35 minutes, until lightly browned, stirring every 5–10 minutes.
4. Allow to cool, then stir in the raisins and coconut. Store in an airtight container and serve with So Good soya milk or soya yogurt.

SERVES 8

PHYTO MUESLI

21/2 mugs puffed rice
2 mugs cornflakes
1/2 mug chopped almonds
1/2 mug pumpkin seeds
1/2 mug chopped pecan nuts

1/2 mug sesame seeds
1/2 mug pine kernels
1/3 mug organic linseeds
2/3 mug organic raisins
1/2 mug organic apricots, chopped

1. Mix the ingredients together and store in a sealed container.
2 Serve with chopped fresh fruit and soya yogurt or So Good.

SERVES 10–12

Note If you are constipated you will need to sprinkle an additional 1–2 tablespoons of organic linseeds on to your muesli each morning for the best results!

SCRAMBLED TOFU

1 tbsp soya oil
1 small onion, finely chopped
1/2 tsp black pepper
1 carrot, finely chopped

medium potato, diced
2 x 275 g (10 oz) cartons plain tofu
1 1/2 tsp turmeric

1. Heat the oil in a large frying pan and sauté the onion until clear and tender. Add the carrot and potato and cook for about 10 minutes, stirring often.
2. Stir in the tofu and turmeric, cover the pan and cook for 5 minutes.
3. Serve hot with toasted rye bread, grilled tomatoes and mushrooms.

SERVES 4

LUNCHES

CARROT AND APRICOT PÂTÉ

75 g (3 oz) organic dried apricots
75 g (3 oz) tofu, mashed
black pepper
25 g (1 oz) ground almonds
1 tbsp lemon juice

75 ml (3 fl oz) water
1 tsp cardamom
1 tsp nutmeg
225 g (8 oz) grated carrot

1. Cut the apricots into small pieces. Place in the water and simmer for 10 minutes or until soft.
2. Mix all the ingredients together by hand including any liquid remaining with the apricots.
3. Place in a small greased loaf tin, cover and bake for 45 minutes at 200°C/400°F/gas mark 6.
4. Cool a little, cut into slices and serve with a salad and rice cakes.

SERVES 4

CARROT AND ALMOND PÂTÉ

225 g (8 oz) carrots, sliced
100 g (4 oz) almonds
1 tsp chopped mint
1 tsp grated orange rind

1 tbsp chopped chives
black pepper
pure orange juice

1. Cook the carrots in a little water until just soft. Sieve and cool.
2. Place the almonds in a food processor and process until finely ground.
3. Add the carrots, mint, orange rind, chives and pepper and process again. If necessary, add a little orange juice to obtain a smooth pâté.

SERVES 4

HUMMUS

225 g (8 oz) chick peas
600 ml (1 pint) water
150 g (5 oz) sesame seeds
2 tbsp (30 ml) tahini

juice of 3 lemons
2 tbsp soya oil
5 garlic cloves
paprika, to taste

1. Soak the chick peas overnight in 600 ml (1 pint) of water. Drain and wash them.
2. Place the chick peas in 600 ml (1 pint) of fresh water, bring to the boil and simmer gently for 2 hours or until tender.
3. Drain the peas.
4. Place the sesame seeds, tahini, garlic, soya oil and half the lemon juice in a blender and reduce to a smooth purée.
5. Add the cooked chick peas a few at a time to the mixture in the blender, add with the remaining lemon juice and blend until smooth.
6. Add a small amount of paprika to produce a spicy taste if required.
7. Serve with rice cakes or buckwheat pancakes.

SERVES 4

BEAN BURGERS

100 g (4 oz) dried beans (butter, soya, black-eyed)
2 garlic cloves, crushed
1 medium onion, finely chopped

2 tomatoes, finely chopped
1 tsp black pepper
1/2 tsp chilli powder
sunflower oil

1. Wash and drain the beans and soak them overnight in fresh water. Drain, rinse and rub the soaked beans to loosen the skins. Rinse again.
2. Cover with fresh water and cook over a medium heat for about 1 hour. Drain the beans and turn into a mixing bowl. Stir in the remaining ingredients and mash the beans to make a thick paste. Form into medium patties.
3. Heat some sunflower oil in a frying pan until piping hot and place the patties in the pan. Fry for about 5 minutes on either side.
4. Serve hot with a salad.

SERVES 4

FRIED TOFU

2 x 275 g (10 oz) blocks plain tofu   4 tbsp sesame oil
4 tbsp cornflour   2 spring onions, finely sliced

1. Cut the tofu into 1-inch cubes and coat in the cornflour. Heat the oil in a frying pan and fry the tofu for about 5 minutes, turning over until all sides are golden brown.
2. Drain the tofu and serve immediately with the spring onion. Serve with a rice salad and dressing of your choice (see p. 223).

POTATO SKINS WITH BROCCOLI AND TOFU FILLING

4 large baking potatoes, scrubbed and scored
225 g (8 oz) broccoli, trimmed and cut into florets
1 tbsp sunflower oil
2 medium onions, chopped
100 g (4 oz) mushrooms, chopped
1 tsp black pepper
1/4 tsp ground nutmeg
275 g (10 oz) firm plain tofu
3 tbsp fresh parsley, finely chopped
1 tbsp mustard

1. Pre-heat the oven to 200°C/400°F/gas mark 6. Bake the potatoes for about 45 minutes, until tender.
2. Steam the broccoli for 12–15 minutes, until just tender, but still bright green.
3. Remove from the pan and leave to one side. Meanwhile, heat the oil in a frying pan and sauté the onions for 5 minutes. Add the mushrooms and sauté over a low heat, stirring often. Add the black pepper and nutmeg and remove from the heat.

4. Slice the baked potatoes in half lengthways and scoop out their insides, leaving a thick shell of potato skin. Combine the potato with the steamed broccoli and the tofu, parsley and mustard in a mixing bowl.

5. Mash these ingredients together to make a smooth mixture. Add the mushrooms and onions and stir well. Spoon this mixture back into the potato skins, letting the filling rise well above the potato shell.

6. Return the potatoes to the oven for 15 minutes. Serve hot with a salad and dressing of your choice.

SERVES 4

BARBECUEd SOYA BEANS

200 g (7 oz) dried soya beans
1 l (2 pints) water
2 tbsp soya oil
2 medium onions, coarsely chopped
2 cloves garlic, crushed
75 g (3 oz) tomato purée
50 g (2 oz) brown sugar
75 ml (3 fl oz) apple cider vinegar
50 ml (2 fl oz) tamari sauce
1 tsp cayenne pepper

1. In a large saucepan, combine the dried soya beans and 600 ml (1 pint) of the water over a high heat. Bring to the boil for 2 minutes, remove from the heat, and let stand for 1 hour. Drain the beans, add the remaining water and cook for 2–3 hours or until the beans are soft.

2. In a separate saucepan, gently heat the oil. Add the onions and garlic, and sauté until tender. Add the tomato purée, brown sugar, apple cider vinegar, tamari and cayenne pepper, and simmer for 20 minutes.

3. Drain the soya beans and add to the mixture; cook for another 30 minutes. Adjust the seasonings, adding more tamari, if necessary.

4. Serve hot with rice or as a filling for a jacket potato.

SERVES 8

BEAN TACOS

75 g (3 oz) textured vegetable protein (TVP)
1 tbsp soya oil
1 medium onion, chopped
1 medium green pepper, finely chopped
2 tbsp tomato purée
400 g (13 oz) tin mixed beans in a spicy sauce

1. Place the TVP in a small bowl and add $1/2$ cup of boiling water. Allow to stand for 10–15 minutes. Rinse and drain well.
2. Heat the oil in a frying pan and gently sauté the onion and pepper until tender. Add the tomato purée, mixed beans and TVP and $1/4$ cup of water. Heat through.
3. Serve the beans in taco shells or over corn chips topped with shredded lettuce, diced tomato and avocado.

SERVES 6

TEMPEH KEBABS WITH PITTA BREAD

2 tsp soya oil
350 g (12 oz) tempeh, finely sliced
4 pitta breads, lightly toasted
8 tbsp hummus (see page 185)
200 g (7 oz) cooked basmati rice

2 medium tomatoes, diced
200 g (7 oz) lettuce, shredded
4 tbsp spicy peanut sauce (see page 226)

1. Heat the oil in a frying pan and add the tempeh and lightly fry on both sides.
2. Spread each pitta bread with 2 tbsp of hummus. Top with the tempeh, rice, tomato, lettuce and peanut sauce.
3. Serve immediately.

SERVES 4

SPICY SOYA BEANS

This recipe can be made in advance, frozen and served for a quick lunch with rice, or as a filling for pancakes or a jacket potato.

450 g (1 lb) dried soya beans, washed and drained
3 bay leaves
2 tbsp soya oil
2 cloves garlic, chopped
1 large onion, chopped
5 cm (2 inch) piece of cinnamon

275 g (10 oz) tomato purée
150 ml (1/4 pint) molasses
150 ml (1/4 pint) prepared mustard
1 l (2 pints) vegetable stock
2 tbsp cider vinegar
1 tbsp tamari sauce

1. Wash the beans and soak them overnight in plenty of fresh water. Drain, rinse well and drain again before cooking for 2–3 hours with the bay leaves until the beans are soft. Remove from the heat and drain away the cooking water.

2. Heat the oil in a saucepan and sauté the garlic and onion until tender. Add the cinnamon and stir for 1 minute. Add the tomato purée, molasses, mustard and stock, stir well and bring to the boil. Add the beans, bring to the boil again then cover the pan, reduce the heat to low and simmer gently for about 1 hour.

3. Stir once during this time and add more stock if necessary. At the end of the cooking time, stir in the vinegar and tamari sauce. Remove the pot from the heat and serve immediately. The beans should be thick and the sauce richly flavoured.

SERVES 6

REFRIED SOYA BEANS

Based on a classic Mexican dish, substituting soya beans for the traditional kidney beans.

1 tbsp soya oil
1 onion, finely chopped
1 clove garlic, crushed

200 g (7 oz) soya beans, washed, cooked in water and drained

1. Fry the onion and garlic in the oil for 2 minutes until lightly browned.
2. Add the cooked soya beans and cook over a gentle heat until warmed through, mashing the beans with a potato masher. Add 1–2 tablespoons water if necessary to prevent sticking.
3. Serve warm with rice and tacos or as a filling for a jacket potato.

SERVES 4

HERBED TOFU PÂTÉ

450 g (1 lb) tofu
1 tbsp tamari sauce
1 tbsp tahini
1 tsp plum sauce

1 tsp fresh lemon juice
1 tbsp chives, finely chopped
1 tbsp fresh basil, finely chopped

1. Place all the ingredients in a food processor and blend until smooth.
2. Press the mixture into a mould and refrigerate overnight until firm.
3. Slice and serve with rice cakes, rye bread and salad.

SERVES 4

TOFU TUNA SPREAD

1 small onion
275 g (10 oz) tofu
175 g (6 oz) tuna
100 g (4 oz) carrots, grated

50 g (2 oz) fresh parsley, chopped
1 tbsp soya mayonnaise
2 tbsp mustard
1 tbsp honey

1. Mince the onion in a food processor. Add the tofu and tuna and process until the mixture is of the desired consistency. Stir in the carrots and parsley.
2. In a small bowl, mix the soya mayonnaise, mustard and honey, then blend into the tuna mixture.

SERVES 4

SOUPS

FENNEL, CELERY AND LEEK SOUP

2 medium leeks
3–4 sticks celery
1 large bulb fennel
1 tsp olive oil
1 tsp fennel seeds

1 tsp celery seeds
600 ml (1 pint) water
300 ml (1/2 pint) So Good soya milk
450 ml (3/4 pint) vegetable stock
black pepper

1. Finely slice the leeks and celery and dice the fennel.
2. Heat the oil in a pan and add the vegetables plus the fennel and celery seeds. Sweat, stirring occasionally, until the vegetables are softened and beginning to brown.
3. Add the water, bring to the boil and simmer for 10 minutes.
4. Allow to cool a little then process until smooth. This stage can be omitted if you prefer a chunky soup or do not have a food processor. Return the mixture to the pan.
5. Add the remaining ingredients and bring to the boil.

SERVES 4

SOYA BEAN AND VEGETABLE SOUP

225 g (8 oz) soya beans
1 l (2 pints) vegetable stock
2 large carrots
1 large parsnip

2 leeks
1/4 tsp dried thyme
black pepper

1. Soak the soya beans overnight.
2. Rinse the beans well and cook in the stock until soft, adding more water if the liquid is evaporating. To save time, use a pressure cooker if available and cook the beans for 10 minutes. The soya beans can be processed at this stage if a smooth soup is required.
3. Grate the carrots and parsnip and place in the pan with the beans.
4. Finely slice the leeks and add to the pan along with the thyme and black pepper. Simmer for 15 minutes and serve.

SERVES 4

LEEK, SWEETCORN AND ALMOND SOUP

1 large onion
700 g (1 1/2 lb) leeks
2 sticks celery
1 tbsp olive oil
75 g (3 oz) whole blanched almonds
900 ml (1 1/2 pints) water

600 ml (1 pint) vegetable stock
175 g (6 oz) sweetcorn kernels
1/2 tsp mustard
1 tbsp fresh parsley
black pepper

1. Chop the onions, leeks and celery then sweat in the oil until the vegetables are soft and beginning to brown.
2. Process the almonds until finely ground, then add half the vegetable mixture and approximately 300 ml (1/2 pint) of water. Process again until smooth and creamy.
3. Return this mixture to the pan along with the remaining ingredients.
4. Bring the soup to the boil and simmer for 10 minutes before serving.

SERVES 4

WATERCRESS SOUP

50 g (2 oz) soya margarine
1 medium onion, finely chopped
225 g (8 oz) potatoes, peeled and
diced
600 ml (1 pint) vegetable stock

pinch of nutmeg
4 bunches of watercress, washed
and trimmed
black pepper, to taste

1. Melt the margarine in a frying pan, add the onion and sweat it gently for about 5 minutes or until the onion is transparent.
2. Add the potatoes, vegetable stock and nutmeg and simmer for 15 minutes.
3. Add the watercress and simmer for a further 10 minutes. Purée the

soup in a blender or food processor, then push through a sieve. Add black pepper to taste and serve straight away.

SERVES 4

POTATO AND BASIL SOUP

1 tbsp soya oil
700 g (11/2 lb) potatoes, peeled and grated
3 garlic cloves, crushed
50 g (2 oz) fresh basil, chopped
900 ml (11/2 pints) vegetable stock
black pepper, to taste

1. Heat the oil in a large saucepan and gently fry the potatoes, garlic and half the basil for 2 minutes, then add the stock.
2. Bring to the boil, then reduce the heat, cover and simmer for 15–20 minutes or until the potatoes are soft.
3. Season with the pepper and mix well or purée in a blender or food processor. Add the remaining basil and serve hot.

SERVES 4

CAULIFLOWER SOUP

50 g (2 oz) soya margarine
100 g (4 oz) soya flour
300 ml (1/2 pint) So Good soya milk
900ml (11/2 pints) vegetable stock
1 large cauliflower, stalk removed
   and broken into florets
1 tsp dried chervil
black pepper, to taste

1. Melt the margarine in a large saucepan. Add the soya flour and cook for 1 minute, stirring constantly. Remove from the heat and gradually stir in the So Good and stock until the mixture is smooth.
2. Add the cauliflower, chervil and black pepper and simmer gently for 15 minutes or until the cauliflower is just soft. Mash the cauliflower well or purée in a blender or food processor, and serve piping hot.

SERVES 4

LENTIL SOUP

100 g (4 oz) split red lentils
1 large onion
1 clove garlic
900 ml (11/2 pints) vegetable stock
1 tsp ground cumin
1 bay leaf
400 g (14 oz) tin chopped tomatoes
1 tsp grated lemon rind
black pepper, to taste

1. Wash the lentils, finely chop the onion and press the garlic.
2. Place all the ingredients in a saucepan and bring to the boil, then simmer for 20–30 minutes.
3. Remove the bay leaf and serve.

SERVES 4

BEAN SOUP

25 g (1 oz) haricot beans
25 g (1 oz) mung beans
25 g (1 oz) aduki beans
25 g (1 oz) soya beans
100 g (4 oz) onion, well chopped

25 g (1 oz) soya oil
black pepper
600 ml (1 pint) vegetable stock
fresh chopped parsley

1. Soak the beans in 600 ml (1 pint) of water overnight. Discard the water and rinse the beans.
2. Cook the onion slowly in the oil for about 10 minutes.
3. Add the beans and the rest of the ingredients.
4. Bring to the boil and boil rapidly for 10 minutes. Then simmer gently for 1^1/2 hours.
5. Serve garnished with fresh chopped parsley.

SERVES 4

POULTRY AND MEAT

CHICKEN AND ALMOND PILAFF

225 g (8 oz) brown rice
175 g (6 oz) cooked chicken
175 g (6 oz) tofu
2 carrots
juice of 1 orange

grated rind of 1/2 orange
3 tbsp organic raisins
black pepper, to taste
100 g (4 oz) toasted flaked almonds

1. Cook the brown rice for about 45 minutes or until tender, and keep warm.
2. Cut the chicken into bite-sized pieces.
3. Sauté the tofu until lightly browned and set aside.
4. Cut the carrots into matchstick pieces.
5. Cook the carrots in the orange juice with the orange rind and raisins for approximately 5 minutes until just cooked. Warm the chicken and the tofu. (NOTE: Ensure that the chicken is thoroughly heated through.)

6. Mix together the rice, chicken, tofu, carrot mixture (including any remaining cooking liquid), the black pepper and the almonds, and serve.

SERVES 4

CHICKEN BURGERS

150 g (5 oz) textured vegetable
protein (TVP)
225 g (8 oz) cooked chicken meat,
minced
1 egg, beaten
1 garlic clove, crushed

1 tbsp finely chopped fresh parsley
2 tsp dried tarragon
black pepper, to taste
1 tbsp soya oil
1 onion, finely chopped

1. Reconstitute the TVP by adding double the volume of water and leave to soak until it has been absorbed. Mix the chicken, TVP and egg together. Add the garlic, parsley, tarragon and pepper, and mix well.
2. Heat the oil in a frying pan and gently fry the onion for 2–3 minutes. Add the onion to the chicken and TVP mixture and stir well.
3. Form the mixture into round burger shapes and place on a greased baking tray.
4. Bake in a pre-heated oven at 180°C/350°F/gas mark 4 for 15–20 minutes or until golden brown, turning once halfway through baking.

SERVES 4

CHICKEN IN SESAME SAUCE

225 g (8 oz) chicken breast
4 tbsp almond butter
3 tbsp soya oil
1 tbsp sesame oil
2 tbsp tamari sauce

3 tbsp sherry
2 tsp sugar
1 pinch cayenne pepper
2 leeks, white part only, finely
chopped

1. Cut the chicken into 2.5 cm (1-inch) cubes.
2. In a small bowl mix together the almond butter, 1 tbsp of the soya oil, sesame oil, tamari and sherry, sugar and cayenne pepper. Set the sauce aside.
3. In a large frying pan, heat the remaining soya oil over a moderate heat. Add the chicken and leeks and cook them for 4 minutes, stirring constantly.
4. Using a slotted spoon, remove the chicken and leeks from the pan.

Drain them on kitchen paper and place them on a heated serving dish. Pour the sauce over the chicken and leeks. Serve with rice and fresh vegetables.

SERVES 2

CHICKEN WITH A YOGURT MARINADE

225 ml (8 fl oz) natural soya
  yogurt
1 tsp curry powder
1/2 bunch coriander, finely chopped

1 tbsp grated fresh root ginger
3 garlic cloves, crushed
chicken, weighing 1–1.5 kg
  (2–4 lb)

1. Combine the soya yogurt, curry powder, coriander, ginger and garlic. Rub all over the chicken and set aside for 1–2 hours.
2. Place the chicken in a roasting tin with the yogurt sauce and bake in a pre-heated oven at 180°C/350°F/gas mark 4 for $1^1/4 –1^1/2$ hours.
3. Transfer the chicken to a serving dish and keep warm. Stir together the chicken juices and yogurt sauce remaining in the roasting tin and boil rapidly to reduce, if necessary. Serve the chicken with the sauce.

SERVES 4

CHICKEN WITH ALMOND SAUCE

2 tbsp soya oil
225 g (8 oz) skinless chicken breast
  fillets, cut into thin strips
225 g (8 oz) tempeh, cut into strips
1 tsp chilli powder

225 g (8 oz) tin tomatoes, finely
  chopped
2 tbsp almond butter
1–2 tsp chilli sauce

1. Heat the oil in a frying pan. Add the chicken and tempeh and stir-fry for 2–3 minutes, sprinkling with the chilli powder while cooking. Remove from the pan with a slotted spoon and set aside.
2. Put the tomatoes, almond butter and chilli sauce into the pan and stir well.
3. Return the chicken and tempeh to the pan and bring to the boil, then reduce the heat and simmer gently, stirring occasionally. Serve immediately.

SERVES 4

LAMB KEBABS WITH MINT YOGURT

450 g (1 lb) lamb fillet
2 tbsp soya oil
2 tbsp orange juice
1 garlic clove, crushed
black pepper, to taste
225 g (8 oz) button onions, skinned
2 courgettes

1 green pepper, de-seeded and cut
  into 2.5 cm (1-inch) pieces
1 red pepper, de-seeded and cut into
  2.5 cm (1-inch) pieces
8 button mushrooms
225 g (8 oz) natural soya yogurt
2 tsp finely chopped mint

1. Cut the lamb into 2.5 cm (1-inch) cubes. Mix the oil, orange juice, garlic and black pepper in shallow dish, add the meat and leave to marinate for 2 hours.
2. Blanch the onions in boiling water for 3 minutes, then drain. Cut the courgettes into 2.5 cm (1-inch) pieces.
3. Drain the lamb, reserving the marinade. Thread the lamb and vegetables on to 8 kebab skewers.
4. Cook under a pre-heated grill for 10–15 minutes, basting occasionally with the marinade.
5. While the kebabs are cooking, prepare the yogurt dressing by mixing the yogurt and mint together.
6. When the kebabs are cooked, serve with the dressing and rice.

SERVES 4

LAMB WITH CRANBERRY SAUCE

4 large boned lamb chops, trimmed
  of excess fat
25 g (1 oz) seasoned flour made
  with 25 g (1 oz) cornflour, pinch
  of cayenne pepper and 1/2 tsp
  dried rosemary

1 tbsp soya margarine
1 tbsp soya oil
4 tbsp tinned cranberries
150 ml (1/4 pint) dry white wine
freshly ground black pepper, to taste
2 tbsp So Good soya milk

1. Dip the chops in the seasoned flour and coat thoroughly on all sides. Shake off any excess flour.
2. Melt the margarine with the oil in a large frying pan. Add the lamb chops and fry for 5 minutes each side, or until they are well browned.
3. Reduce the heat and continue cooking the chops for 20–30 minutes or until they are thoroughly cooked and tender.
4. Transfer the lamb to a warmed serving dish and keep the chops hot while you make the sauce.
5. Remove the frying pan from the heat and pour off all the fat except 1 tablespoon.

6. Return the pan to the heat and stir in the cranberries, wine and pepper. Bring to the boil. Cook the sauce for 5 minutes, stirring occasionally.
7. Stir in the So Good and pour the sauce over the chops. Serve immediately.

SERVES 4

LAMB STIR-FRY WITH ALMONDS AND WALNUTS

6 dried apricots
350 g (12 oz) tender loin organic
   lamb
2 tsp cornflour
4 tbsp water
4 tbsp orange juice
2 tsp soya oil

4 spring onions, cut diagonally into
   2.5 cm (1-inch) pieces
1 tbsp tamari sauce
3 medium Chinese leaves, roughly
   chopped
50 g (2 oz) walnut pieces
black pepper, to taste

1. Soak the apricots in cold water for about 1 hour, then drain and cut them into quarters.
2. Remove any fat from the lamb and cut into very thin strips.
3. Blend the cornflour with 1 tablespoon of water, then add the rest of the water and the orange juice.
4. Heat the oil in a frying pan or wok. Add the lamb and stir-fry for 3–4 minutes or until browned. Reduce the heat to moderate, add the spring onions, tamari sauce and Chinese leaves, and continue to stir-fry for a further minute.
5. Add the apricots and cornflour mixture to the pan and bring to the boil over a moderate to high heat, stirring constantly. After about 30 seconds, the mixture should become thick and glossy.
6. Remove the pan from the heat and stir in the walnuts. Season with pepper and serve with rice and vegetables.

SERVES 4

LAMB CHOPS WITH ROSEMARY

3 tbsp soya oil
2 tbsp lemon juice
freshly ground black pepper, to taste

2 tsp dried rosemary
1 garlic clove, crushed
4 thick boned lamb chops

1. In a medium sized shallow mixing bowl combine the oil, lemon juice, pepper, rosemary and garlic.

2. Place the lamb chops in the marinade and baste them well. Set aside in a cool place and marinate for 1–2 hours, basting frequently.
3. Pre-heat the grill to high. Place the lamb chops on the grill rack. Reserve the marinade. Grill the chops for 2 minutes on each side, basting them frequently with the marinade, or until they are tender when pierced with the point of a sharp knife.
4. Remove the chops from the grill and place them on a warmed serving plate. Spoon the warmed marinade over the chops and serve immediately.

SERVES 4

LAMB STEAKS IN POMEGRANATE AND WALNUT SAUCE

2 tbsp soya oil
1 large onion, finely chopped
350 g (12 oz) walnuts, crushed
black pepper to taste
1 tsp ground cinnamon
1 tsp ground coriander
3 tbsp tomato purée

900 ml (1 1/2 pints) vegetable stock
juice of 2 lemons
4 tbsp grenadine (pomegranate syrup)
4 lamb steaks (boneless)
1 fresh pomegranate, quartered and deseeded (retain the seeds)

1. Heat 1 tablespoon of the oil in a large saucepan and sauté the onion over a medium heat, until clear and tender. Add the walnuts and sauté for a further 5 minutes, stirring constantly.
2. Add the spices and stir for 1 minute. Stir in the tomato purée and stock and bring to the boil. Cover the pan, reduce the heat and leave to simmer for 20 minutes.
3. Add the lemon juice and grenadine and more stock if necessary, stir well. Put the sauce to one side while you prepare the lamb.
4. Sauté the lamb in the remaining oil until well browned. Add the sauce to the pan and cover, simmering for about 10 minutes.
5. Serve the lamb over rice, cover with the sauce and garnish with a few pomegranate seeds.

SERVES 4

FISH AND SHELLFISH

BAKED AVOCADO WITH TUNA

25 g (1 oz) soya margarine
50 g (2 oz) soya flour
150 ml (1/4 pint) So Good soya milk
black pepper, to taste
100 g (4 oz) tin tuna chunks in
  soya oil, drained and flaked

1 tbsp lemon juice
2 large ripe avocados
25 g (1 oz) Gruyère cheese, grated
lemon slices

1. Melt the margarine in a saucepan, stir in the soya flour and cook for 1¹/2 minutes, stirring constantly.
2. Remove from the heat and gradually stir in the So Good. Bring slowly to the boil, stirring constantly, then simmer for 2 minutes, stirring until thickened. Season with pepper and remove from the heat.
3. Stir the tuna and lemon juice into the sauce, being careful not to break up the tuna.
4. Cut the avocados in half and remove the stones. Stand the avocado halves in a baking dish, using crumpled foil, if necessary, to help them stand upright.
5. Spoon the tuna mixture on to the avocados, covering all the avocado flesh. Sprinkle with the grated cheese and bake in a pre-heated oven at 180°C/350°F/gas mark 4 for 15–20 minutes.
6. Transfer the avocados to serving dishes, garnish with lemon slices and serve immediately.

SERVES 4

PRAWN CURRY

1 tbsp soya oil
1 medium onion, chopped
2 garlic cloves, crushed
1 tbsp soya flour
2 tsp curry powder

475 ml (16 fl oz) water
1 tbsp tomato purée
1 medium potato, peeled and sliced
275 g (10 oz) peeled cooked prawns

1. Heat the oil in a frying pan and gently fry the onion and garlic for 2–3 minutes.
2. Add the soya flour and curry powder, mix well and cook, stirring for 1 minute.
3. Add the water and tomato purée and continue to cook, stirring,

until the mixture thickens. Add the potato, cover and simmer for 15 minutes.

4. Add the prawns and simmer for a further 5 minutes or until the potato is tender. Serve with rice or spinach pasta.

SERVES 4

SALMON STEAKS WITH GINGER

2 salmon steaks
2 tbsp lemon juice
2.5 cm (1-inch) square of fresh root
  ginger, peeled and finely chopped

black pepper, to taste

1. Place each salmon steak on a large piece of foil. Add 1 tablespoon of lemon juice and half the chopped ginger to each steak. Season with a little black pepper.

2. Wrap the steaks individually in foil to make two parcels and bake in a pre-heated oven at 180°C/350°F/gas mark 4 for 20 minutes. Serve hot with vegetables or cold with a salad.

SERVES 2

SALMON POTATO CAKES

450 g (1 lb) tin salmon
200 g (7 oz) potatoes, coarsely
  grated

1 egg, lightly beaten
3 green shallots, sliced
2 tsp soya oil

1. Drain the salmon and reserve the liquid. Remove the bones and skin.

2. Place the salmon in a bowl and mix in the potatoes, egg and shallots. Divide the mixture into 8 portions and pat into the desired shape.

3. Heat the oil in a frying pan, add the salmon potato cakes and fry on each side until golden brown. Serve with any sauce from the Sauces and Dressings section (see page 223).

SERVES 4

QUICK PRAWN AND ALMOND RISOTTO

1 tbsp soya oil
4 leeks, chopped
1 red pepper, de-seeded and chopped
100 g (4 oz) brown long-grain rice,
  cooked
100 g (4 oz) frozen peas
100 g (4 oz) frozen sweetcorn

1 tsp grated orange rind
1/2 tsp cayenne pepper
1/2 tsp ground cumin
black pepper, to taste
225 g (8 oz) prawns
100 g (4 oz) almonds

1. Heat the oil in a large saucepan and sauté the leeks and red pepper until soft.
2. Add the rice, vegetables and orange rind and heat through thoroughly, for about 20 minutes.
3. Stir in the seasoning, prawns and almonds. Serve immediately with a green salad.

SERVES 4

TUNA AND LENTIL BAKE

175 g (6 oz) split red lentils
600 ml (1 pint) water
1 large onion, diced
1 tbsp soya oil
2 large eggs

150 ml (1/4 pint) So Good soya milk
200 g (7 oz) tuna chunks in soya
  oil
black pepper, to taste
2 tbsp chopped nuts

1. Wash the lentils and bring to the boil in a pan with 600 ml (1 pint) water. Simmer for 20–25 minutes until the lentils are soft and most of the liquid has been absorbed.
2. Sweat the onion in the oil until it begins to soften.
3. Separate the eggs and beat the yolks and So Good together. Whisk the egg whites until stiff.
4. Flake the tuna fish and include the juices from the tin.
5. Combine the lentils, onion, tuna, egg, So Good and black pepper. Fold in the egg whites using a metal spoon.
6. Pour the mixture into a shallow, greased ovenproof dish, sprinkle the surface with the nuts and bake at 180°C/350°F/gas mark 4 for 30 minutes or until it is set and brown.

SERVES 4

SALMON STUFFED COURGETTES

4 large courgettes　　　　　　　50 g (2 oz) soya cream 'cheese'
100 g (4 oz) cooked, flaked salmon　black pepper

1. Blanch the courgettes in boiling water for 10 minutes. Lift out and leave to cool.
2. When cold, halve the courgettes lengthways and spoon out the centres. Chop finely and mix with the salmon, 'cheese' and pepper. Pile the stuffing back into the shells and place under a hot grill for 10 minutes until lightly browned.
3. Serve with a jacket potato and orange and avocado salad (see p. 221).

SERVES 4

FISH AND RICE BAKE

100 g (4 oz) long-grain rice
450 g (1 lb) cod or haddock
350 ml (3/4 pint) So Good soya
　milk
225 g (8 oz) prawns
25 g (1 oz) soya margarine

25 g (1 oz) soya flour
100 g (4 oz) Cheddar cheese,
　grated
black pepper
4 eggs
2 tbsp chopped fresh parsley

1. Cook the rice according to the packet, rinse and drain well.
2. Cook the fish gently in half the So Good in a covered pan. When cooked, remove the fish and reserve the liquid. Mix the fish, prawns and rice together and put into an ovenproof dish. Stir in the chopped parsley.
3. Melt the margarine in a saucepan, stir in the soya flour until a thick paste is produced. Remove from the heat and mix in the remaining So Good and reserved liquid to make the sauce. Add three-quarters of the cheese and pepper and mix well.
4. Mix the cheese sauce into the fish and rice and sprinkle with the remaining cheese.
5. Bake in a pre-heated oven at 180°C/350°F/gas mark 4 for about 20 minutes until the top turns golden brown.
6. While the casserole is cooking, poach the eggs and place on top of the fish when it comes out of the oven. Garnish with fresh parsley.

SERVES 4

COD WITH ORANGE AND ALMONDS

50 g (2 oz) soya margarine
75 g (3 oz) fresh brown breadcrumbs*
1 garlic clove, finely chopped
50 g (2 oz) almonds, finely chopped

finely grated peel and juice of
  1 medium orange
4 cod cutlets, bones removed
black pepper

1. Melt the margarine in a pan and stir in the breadcrumbs, garlic, almonds and orange peel. Leave over a low heat, stirring frequently until the margarine has been absorbed by the crumbs.
2. Sprinkle the fish with black pepper. Stand the cutlets in an oven-proof dish, pour over the orange juice and cover with the breadcrumbs mixture.
3. Bake uncovered in a pre-heated oven at 180°C/350°F/gas mark 4 for 20–30 minutes until the fish is tender.

SERVES 4

*If you are following a gluten/wheat free diet use an alternative bread.

VEGETARIAN OPTIONS

CARROT AND COURGETTE BAKE

1 onion, diced
1 tbsp soya oil
2 courgettes, grated
2 carrots, grated
2 eggs
25 g (1 oz) rice flour

50 g (2 oz) soya flour
100 ml (4 fl oz) So Good soya milk
1/2 tsp potassium-rich baking powder
1/2 tsp dried rosemary
1/2 tsp dried thyme
black pepper

1. Sweat the onion in the soya oil until it begins to soften but remains colourless.
2. In a bowl mix the onion, courgettes and carrots.
3. Beat the eggs with the rice flour, soya flour, So Good, baking powder, herbs and black pepper. Combine the two mixtures.
4. Pour into a greased gratin dish and bake uncovered at 200°C/400°F/gas mark 6 for 45 minutes to 1 hour or until brown and set. Serve with baked potatoes and a selection of salads.

SERVES 4

BEAN AND TOFU CASSEROLE

1 whole corn on the cob
1 large parsnip
2 carrots
1/2 small swede
2 medium onions
2 courgettes
175 g (6 oz) plain tofu
225 g (8 oz) cooked kidney beans

1/2 tsp dried thyme
1/2 tsp dried rosemary
1 bay leaf
black pepper
450 ml (3/4 pint) water
300 ml (1/2 pint) So Good soya
  milk
2 level tbsp cornflour

1. Cut the corn on the cob into 1.5 cm (^{1}/2–inch) sections.
2. Cut the remaining vegetables into chunks, adjusting the size according to how quickly they cook. Place all the vegetables into a casserole dish.
3. Cube the tofu and add to the casserole along with the kidney beans, herbs, pepper and water. Mix gently.
4. Cover the casserole and cook for 1 hour at 200°C/400°F/gas mark 6. There should be only a small amount of liquid left in the casserole but watch to make sure it does not dry up altogether.
5. When cooked, lift out the vegetables and tofu using a slotted spoon, and remove the bay leaf.
6. Mix the So Good to a smooth paste with the cornflour and add to the juices in the casserole dish. Bring to the boil on top of the cooker, stirring constantly, and simmer for 2 minutes. Return the vegetables to the pan and gently mix.

SERVES 4

BROCCOLI AND SMOKED TOFU BAKE

1 medium onion
225 g (8 oz) broccoli florets
300 ml (1/2 pint) water
2 level tbsp soya flour
300 ml (1/2 pint) So Good soya milk
1/4 tsp nutmeg
1/2 tsp lemon rind
black pepper
225 g (8 oz) cooked red kidney
  beans
225 g (8 oz) smoked tofu, cubed

Topping:
75 g (3 oz) millet flakes
25 g (1 oz) brown rice flour
50 g (2 oz) ground nuts, e.g.
  almonds, hazelnuts
2 tbsp soya oil
2 tbsp sunflower seeds

1. Chop the onion and cook with the broccoli in 150 ml ($^1/4$ pint) boiling water until just tender. Drain and keep the cooking liquid.
2. Put the soya flour in a pan and mix to a smooth paste using a little of the So Good. Add the remaining So Good and the stock from the vegetables made up to 150 ml ($^1/4$ pint) with water.
3. Bring to the boil, stirring constantly, then lower the heat and simmer for 2 minutes.
4. Add the nutmeg, lemon rind and pepper, then the onion and broccoli, beans and tofu.
5. Spoon the mixture into a large gratin dish (or 4 small dishes).
6. To make the topping, place the millet flakes, rice flour and ground nuts in a bowl and rub in the oil by hand.
7. Spread the topping over the vegetable and tofu mixture and scatter the sunflower seeds over the surface.

SERVES 4

BARLEY ROAST WITH TAHINI SAUCE

1 tbsp soya oil	450 g (1 lb) barley, thoroughly
1 medium onion, chopped	cooked
1 medium carrot, chopped	black pepper
1 large green pepper	200 g (7 oz) Cheddar cheese, grated
225 g (8 oz) mushrooms	2 eggs, beaten
1 tbsp tamari sauce	1 large tomato, sliced
3 sprigs parsley, chopped	tahini sauce (see page 206)

1. Heat the oil in a pan. Stir-fry the onions and carrots. When the onion softens add the rest of the vegetables.
2. When all the vegetables are hot, add the tamari sauce and parsley. Remove from the heat.
3. Stir in the barley and adjust the seasoning.
4. Add 125 g (4 oz) of the cheese and the eggs. If the mixture is too dry add a little vegetable stock. Pour the mixture into a greased and lined 900 g (2 lb) loaf tin.
5. Sprinkle the top with the remaining cheese and decorate with slices of tomato. Bake in a moderate oven for 35 minutes until well browned.
6. Serve with tahini sauce.

SERVES 4

TAHINI SAUCE

50 g (2 oz) soya margarine
50 g (2 oz) soya flour
600 ml (1 pint) So Good soya milk
1 large onion, finely sliced
1 bay leaf

100 ml (4 fl oz) tahini
3 cloves garlic, crushed
juice of 1 lemon
black pepper, to taste

1. Melt the margarine in a pan and add the soya flour. Allow to cook until a light creamy colour is achieved. Allow to cool.
2. Boil the So Good with the onion and bay leaf. Gradually add to the flour and fat mixture, stirring continuously with a wooden spoon until smooth and lump free.
3. Add the tahini, garlic and lemon juice, and stir well until combined. Season with black pepper to taste.

SHEPHERDESS PIE

50 ml (2 fl oz) soya oil
1 medium onion, sliced
1 medium carrot, sliced
1 small parsnip, chopped
1 small swede, chopped
1 bunch parsley, chopped
1 tbsp tamari sauce
450 g (1 lb) leeks

300 ml (1/2 pint) tahini sauce (see above) (tahini omitted)
225 g (8 oz) aduki beans, cooked
450 g (1 lb) potatoes, cooked and mashed
100 g (4 oz) Cheddar cheese, grated
black pepper to taste

1. Heat the oil and stir-fry the root vegetables with the parsley until quite hot. Add the tamari sauce, season and add the leeks. Cook for another 5 minutes on a medium heat. Remove from the heat.
2. Add the tahini sauce to the vegetables, then stir in the aduki beans. Adjust seasoning and turn the ingredients into an ovenproof dish.
3. Spread the mashed potatoes evenly over the surface.
4. Sprinkle over the cheese and bake in the oven at 180°C/350°F/gas mark 4, for about 10 minutes or until the potatoes have browned.

SERVES 4

TOFU, BEAN AND HERB STIR-FRY

2 tbsp soya oil
275 g (10 oz) tofu, drained, dried
  and cut into cubes
2 garlic cloves, crushed
350 g (12 oz) green beans

3 tbsp chopped fresh herbs (thyme,
  parsley, chervil and chives)
4 spring onions, thinly sliced
2 tbsp tamari sauce

1. Heat 1 tablespoon of the soya oil in a frying pan or wok.
2. When the oil is hot, add the tofu and garlic and stir-fry for 2 minutes. Lift out with a slotted spoon and drain.
3. Heat the remaining oil in the pan and, when hot, add the green beans and stir-fry gently for 4–5 minutes.
4. Add the herbs, spring onions and tamari sauce, and stir-fry for a further minute.
5. Return the tofu to the pan and heat thoroughly for 1 minute, then serve immediately, with rice or noodles.

SERVES 4

COURGETTE AND TOMATO QUICHE

225 g (8 oz) shortcrust
  pastry/wheat-free variation (see
  Pastry section on page 245)
50 g (2 oz) soya margarine
2 garlic cloves, crushed
4 courgettes, trimmed and sliced
freshly ground black pepper, to taste

1/2 tsp oregano
100 ml (4 fl oz) So Good soya milk
3 eggs
50 g (2 oz) Cheddar cheese, grated
5 small tomatoes, peeled and thinly
  sliced

1. Line a flan dish with the pastry and set aside.
2. Pre-heat the oven to 200°C/400°F/gas mark 6.
3. Melt the margarine in a large frying pan. Add the garlic and fry, stirring frequently, for 1 minute.
4. Add the courgettes and pepper. Fry for 8–10 minutes or until lightly browned.
5. Remove the pan from the heat and add the oregano, mixing well to blend.
6. In a mixing bowl, combine the So Good, eggs and cheese. Beat well to blend.

7. Arrange the courgettes and tomatoes in circles in the pastry flan case.
8. Pour the egg, So Good and cheese mixture over the courgettes and tomatoes.
9. Place in the centre of the oven and bake for 35–45 minutes or until the filling is set and golden brown.

SERVES 4–6

SPINACH GRATIN

2 slices of dry bread
50 g (2 oz) Cheddar cheese
450 g (1 lb) fresh or frozen
   spinach, cooked and drained well

1/2 tsp grated nutmeg
freshly ground black pepper

1. Pre-heat the oven to 230°C/450°F/gas mark 8.
2. Break up the bread into rough breadcrumbs.
3. Grate the cheese.
4. Mix the spinach with the nutmeg, add pepper to taste and half the grated cheese, and place in an ovenproof dish.
5. Mix the remaining cheese with the breadcrumbs and sprinkle them over the top.
6. Bake for about 15 minutes until golden brown.

SERVES 4

LEEK GRATIN

1 tbsp soya oil
1 onion, finely chopped
2 garlic cloves, crushed
275 g (10 oz) button mushrooms
4 small courgettes, roughly
   chopped
100 g (4 oz) fresh white
   breadcrumbs
1 tbsp tomato purée
black pepper, to taste

3 large leeks, sliced
100 g (4 oz) French beans

Cheese Sauce
25 g (1 oz) soya margarine
2 tbsp soya flour
450 ml (3/4 pint) So Good soya
   milk
100 g (4 oz) Cheddar cheese
black pepper, to taste

1. Heat the oil in a frying pan and gently fry the onion and garlic for 2–3 minutes.

2. Add the mushrooms and courgettes and cook for a further 2 minutes. Stir in the breadcrumbs, tomato purée and black pepper, then remove from the heat and cover.
3. Cook the leeks and French beans in boiling water for 15 minutes or until just tender. Drain, place in an ovenproof dish and cover with the mushroom mixture.
4. Make the cheese sauce: melt the margarine in a saucepan. Add the soya flour and cook over a low heat, stirring for 1 minute.
5. Remove from the heat and gradually stir in the So Good. Return to the heat and slowly bring back to the boil, stirring constantly. Simmer for a further 2 minutes or until the sauce is thick and smooth.
6. Stir in the cheese and season with pepper. Heat gently without boiling.
7. Pour the cheese sauce over the leek and mushroom mixture. Sprinkle with the cheese and bake in a pre-heated oven at 200°C/400°F/gas mark 6 for 20 minutes.

SERVES 4–6

LENTIL BOLOGNESE

100 g (4 oz) brown lentils	1 tsp dried oregano
1 onion	1 tsp dried basil
1/2 green pepper	600 ml (1 pint) tomato passata
1 stick celery	(finely sieved tomatoes)
1 carrot	1 bay leaf
1 clove garlic	black pepper, to taste
300 ml (1/2 pint) water	

1. Wash the lentils well.
2. Finely chop the onion, green pepper and celery. Dice the carrot and press the garlic clove.
3. Place all the ingredients in a pan, bring to the boil and simmer covered, for 30 minutes or until lentils are soft but not mushy.

SERVES 4

INDONESIAN TOFU KEBABS WITH SATAY SAUCE

275 g (10 oz) plain tofu cut into	1 tbsp soya oil
2.5-cm (1-inch) dice	1 garlic clove, crushed
2 tbsp tamari sauce	4 shallots, halved
1 tbsp honey	1 red pepper, cut into small chunks

Sauce
1 tbsp soya oil
1 shallot, finely chopped
1 green chilli, de-seeded and finely
  chopped
1/4 tsp cumin

1/4 tsp cayenne pepper
50 g (2 oz) creamed coconut
4 tbsp crunchy peanut butter
1 tbsp tamari sauce
150 ml (1/4 pint) boiling water

1. Marinate the tofu in 1 tablespoon tamari sauce for 30 minutes.
2. Make a flavoured oil with the remaining tamari sauce, honey, oil and garlic.
3. Prepare the sauce by heating the oil and frying the shallot, chilli, cumin and cayenne for 3 minutes.
4. Dissolve the coconut in boiling water and add to the pan along with the peanut butter and tamari sauce, mix and cook for 3–4 minutes.
5. Baste the kebabs with the flavoured oil and place under a medium grill for 10 minutes, turning frequently, until browned. Serve with rice and the satay sauce.

SERVES 2

RED LENTIL DHAL

450 g (1 lb) red lentils, washed and
  drained
1 l (2 pints) water
1 tsp salt
2 tbsp soya oil
5 garlic cloves, crushed

1 medium onion, finely chopped
1 tbsp cumin
1 tsp turmeric
1/4–1/2 tsp chilli powder
2 tbsp garam masala
50 g (2 oz) fresh coriander

1. Put washed lentils into a deep saucepan and add the water and salt. Place over a medium heat, bring to the boil and remove some of the froth with a large spoon. Cover the pan, reduce the heat and leave to simmer for about 25 minutes, stirring occasionally. The lentils are cooked when they lose their shape and begin to soften.
2. Heat the oil in a frying pan and sauté the garlic and onion until clear and tender, about 10 minutes. Add the cumin and turmeric and stir over a medium heat for 1–2 minutes, until it has turned golden. Add the chilli powder and stir for a further 1 minute. Turn the sautéed onion and garlic into the cooked lentils and stir well. Allow to simmer for a further 5 minutes. Remove the lentils from the heat, stir in the garam masala and chopped coriander and serve immediately over steamed rice or as a dip with *crudités* and corn chips.

SERVES 4

NOODLES IN SPICY SESAME SAUCE

450 g (1 lb) rice noodles
150 ml (1/4 pint) sesame oil
3 cloves garlic, finely chopped
2 tbsp fresh ginger, finely grated
5 spring onions, finely chopped
black pepper, to taste
1 tsp chilli powder

150 ml (1/4 pint) tahini
2 tbsp tamari sauce
3 tbsp rice vinegar
1 tbsp tomato purée
150 ml (1/4 pint) cold water
1–2 tomatoes, finely chopped

1. Bring a large pot of salted water to the boil and drop in the noodles. Leave until cooked (about 5 minutes).
2. Heat the oil in a frying pan or wok and sauté the garlic and ginger, stirring constantly for 3 minutes over a medium heat. Add the onions and sauté for a further 3 minutes. Add the pepper and chilli and sauté for 1 minute.
3. Blend the remaining ingredients, except the chopped tomatoes, together in a jug and add to the sautéed mixture. Stir well and simmer, cover the pan and remove it from the heat.
4. When the noodles are soft, turn into a serving dish and spoon the sauce over, garnished with the chopped tomatoes.

SERVES 4

SOYA FELAFEL WITH SESAME YOGURT DRESSING

450 g (14 oz) soya beans, soaked, cooked and drained
6 spring onions, finely chopped
25 g (1 oz) white breadcrumbs
1 egg, lightly beaten
grated zest and juice of one lemon
1 garlic clove, crushed
2 tbsp fresh coriander
2 tbsp fresh parsley
1 tbsp tahini paste
1 tsp ground coriander
1 tsp ground cumin

1/2 tsp ground cinnamon
pinch of cayenne pepper
salt and black pepper, to taste
soya oil for deep frying

Dressing
4 tbsp natural soya yogurt
2 tbsp soya oil
1 tbsp lemon juice
1 tbsp tahini paste
salt and black pepper, to taste

1. In a food processor, purée the soya beans, spring onions, breadcrumbs, egg, lemon zest and juice, garlic, coriander, parsley, tahini, ground coriander, cumin, cinnamon, cayenne pepper, and salt and pepper to taste until smooth.

211

2. Turn into a bowl, cover, and leave to stand for at least 30 minutes.
3. Meanwhile, make the sesame dressing: in a bowl, combine the soya yogurt, oil, lemon juice, tahini, and salt and pepper to taste. Cover and set aside.
4. Shape the felafel mixture into balls about the size of walnuts, then flatten them into patties.
5. In a deep fat fryer, heat the oil to 190°C (375°F)*. Lower the felafel into the fryer in batches and cook for 2–3 minutes until golden. Lift out and drain on paper towels. Serve warm with pitta bread, and the sesame yogurt dressing.

SERVES 4–6

*Ensure the fat reaches this temperature so that a minimum amount is absorbed during cooking.

STUFFED BAKED PEPPERS

275 g (10 oz) plain tofu, diced into 1.5 cm (1/2-inch) cubes
50 g (2 oz) sultanas
1 tbsp sherry
2 tbsp tamari sauce
75 g (3 oz) basmati rice
1 small onion, finely chopped
1 tbsp soya oil
4 medium red peppers
25 g (1 oz) almonds, chopped
2 tbsp fresh parsley, chopped
black pepper

1. Place the cubed tofu, sultanas, sherry and tamari sauce in a bowl, mix well and leave to soak.
2. Cook the rice according to the packet (approximately 12 minutes).
3. In a saucepan gently sauté the onion in the soya oil for about 5 minutes.
4. Pre-heat the oven to 190°C/375°F/gas mark 5. Halve the peppers lengthways, remove the pips and pith and leave the stalks intact. Brush the outer skin with soya oil, and arrange on a baking tray ready to fill.
5. Once the rice is cooked, drain thoroughly. In a large bowl mix the rice, cooked onion, soaked tofu and sultanas, almonds, parsley and black pepper.
6. Divide the mixture between the pepper halves, filling generously.
7. Loosely cover the tray of peppers with foil. Place in the oven and bake for about 35 minutes. Remove the foil and place under a hot grill until well browned.

SERVES 4

'LASAGNE'

100 g (4 oz) textured vegetable
   protein (TVP) mince
600 ml (1 pint) water
1 onion, diced
2 garlic cloves, crushed
1 tbsp soya oil
450 g (14 oz) tin chopped tomatoes
300 ml (1/2 pint) passata
2 tbsp red wine
75 g (3 oz) mushrooms, sliced
1 tsp paprika
1 tsp oregano
4 bay leaves
1 tsp sugar
1 tsp basil
black pepper
1 packet pre-cooked lasagne*

Cheese sauce
50 g (2 oz) soya margarine
1 tbsp cornflour
600 ml (1 pint) So Good soya
   milk
75 g (3 oz) Cheddar cheese,
   grated
black pepper

1. Reconstitute the TVP by adding the water and leaving to stand until absorbed.
2. Pre-heat the oven to 200°C/400°F/gas mark 6. Gently sauté the onion and garlic in the oil until tender. Stir in the tomatoes, passata and red wine.
3. Add all the other ingredients (except the lasagne), including the TVP and simmer gently for 15 minutes.
4. Make the cheese sauce; melt the margarine in a saucepan. Add the cornflour and cook over a low heat, stirring for 1 minute. Remove from the heat and gradually stir in the So Good. Return to the heat and slowly bring back to the boil, stirring constantly. Simmer for a further 2 minutes or until the sauce is thick and smooth. Stir in 50 g (2 oz) of the cheese. Add the pepper and stir again.
5. In an ovenproof dish layer the 'meat' sauce with the lasagne sheets and cheese sauce ending with a layer of sauce. Sprinkle the remaining cheese over and bake for about 30 minutes. Serve with a green salad.

SERVES 4

*If you are following a gluten/wheat-free diet you can omit the lasagne and substitute corn pasta or use as a 'Bolognese' sauce.

MARINATED TEMPEH

2 x 225 g (8 oz) blocks tempeh
3 cloves garlic, finely chopped
2 medium onions, chopped
1 apple, quartered, cored and
   chopped
200 ml (7 fl oz) sesame oil
200 ml (7 fl oz) cider vinegar

juice of 2 lemons
50 ml (2 fl oz) tamari sauce
25 g (1 oz) fresh ginger, sliced
2 tsp black peppercorns, crushed
12 whole cloves
7.5-cm (3-inch) piece of cinnamon

1. Cut the tempeh into 2.5 cm (1-inch) cubes and arrange in an oven-proof dish. Mix the remaining ingredients together in a large jug. Stir well then pour over the tempeh.
2. Cover the dish and leave to marinate for 6–8 hours, or overnight.
3. Pre-heat the oven to 190°C/375°F/gas mark 5 and bake the tempeh for 1 hour.
4. Serve hot with stir-fried mixed vegetables and rice or rice noodles.

SERVES 4

SPICY CHILLI

100 g (4 oz) TVP mince
600 ml (1 pint) water
1 tbsp soya oil
3 cloves garlic, finely chopped
2 medium onions, thinly sliced
1 tsp chilli powder
150 g (5 oz) tomato purée

400 g (14 oz) tin chopped tomatoes
1 whole red chilli
225 g (8 oz) cooked soya beans
225 g (8 oz) cooked red kidney
   beans
2 tsp tamari sauce
1 tbsp cider vinegar

1. Reconstitute the TVP by adding the water and leaving to stand until absorbed.
2. Heat the oil in a saucepan and sweat the garlic and onions until clear and tender. Add the chilli powder and sauté for a further 1 minute. Stir in the reconstituted TVP, then the tomato purée and chopped tomatoes. Stir well and leave to simmer over a medium heat.
3. Add the whole chilli and the soya and kidney beans. Add more water at this stage if necessary. Cover the pan, reduce the heat and leave to simmer for about 20 minutes. Add the tamari sauce and cider vinegar 5 minutes before serving. Serve piping hot with rice and tortilla chips.

SERVES 4

SOYA BEAN CASSEROLE

1 tbsp soya oil
1 large onion, peeled and sliced
2 sticks of celery, chopped
100 g (4 oz) carrots, chopped
175 g (6 oz) savoy cabbage,
  chopped
400 g (14 oz) tinned plum
  tomatoes, chopped

1 tbsp tomato purée
1/2 tsp ginger
225 g (8 oz) soya beans soaked,
  cooked in water and drained
50 g (2 oz) cashew nuts
black pepper, to taste

1. Heat the oil in a frying pan and gently fry the onion for 2–3 minutes. Add the carrots and celery and cook for a further 3 minutes.
2. Add the cabbage, tomatoes, tomato purée and ginger and simmer for 10 minutes.
3. Add the cooked soya beans, cashew nuts and black pepper and simmer for a further 5 minutes before serving.

SERVES 4

SOYA BEAN BIRYANI

1 tbsp soya oil
1 medium onion, finely
  chopped
200 g (7 oz) long-grain rice
2 tsp curry powder, hot, medium or
  mild to taste
water
1 large red pepper, seeded and
  diced
1 medium aubergine, diced

2 tsp of caraway seeds
1/2 tsp finely chopped red chilli
  pepper
4 cardamom pods
400 g (14 oz) tin tomatoes
175 g (6 oz) soya beans,
  soaked, cooked in water
  and drained
4 tbsp tinned sweetcorn

1. Heat the oil in a large saucepan and cook the onion for 2–3 minutes. Add the rice and cook for a further 2 minutes.
2. Mix the curry powder with a tablespoon of water and add to the rice. Then add the red pepper, aubergine, caraway seeds, chilli pepper and cardamom pods and stir well over a low heat for a further 2 minutes.
3. Drain the tomatoes, keep the juice to one side and add the tomatoes, chopped, to the rice mixture.
4. Make the tomato juice up to 600 ml (1 pint) with water and add to the rice mixture. Cover and simmer for 20 minutes. Then add

the soya beans and sweetcorn, cover and continue to simmer for a further 10 to 15 minutes, until the rice is cooked.
5. Remove cardamom pods before serving.

SERVES 4

ITALIAN CORN PASTA

100 g (4 oz) textured vegetable protein (TVP) mince
200 ml (7 fl oz) vegetable stock
tomato sauce (see below)
275 g (10 oz) corn pasta
50 g (2 oz) grated vegetarian cheese
4 sprigs of parsley to garnish

Tomato sauce
2 tsp soya oil

100 g (4 oz) onion, finely chopped
1 clove garlic, crushed
400 g (14 oz) fresh ripe tomatoes, chopped and skin removed, or 400 g (14 oz) tin plum tomatoes, drained and chopped
mixed herbs or basil
freshly ground black pepper, to taste

1. To make the sauce: heat the oil, add the onion and garlic, cover, and cook gently for 5 minutes until the onion is soft.
2. Add the tomatoes and herbs. Cover and cook for 15 minutes.
3. Season with freshly ground black pepper.
4. Cook the TVP mince in vegetable stock together with the tomato sauce. Simmer for 10 minutes.
5. Cook the pasta in boiling water as directed on the packet.
6. Drain the pasta and divide into 4 dishes and pour the sauce over the pasta. Top with grated cheese and sprigs of parsley.

SERVES 4

NUTTY TEMPEH STIR-FRY

75 g (3 oz) unsalted peanuts
1 tbsp soya oil
200 g (7 oz) tempeh
1 medium orange, peeled and cut into segments
1 pinch of cayenne
1/2 tsp ground cumin seeds
2 thick spring onions, trimmed and sliced

1 garlic clove, thinly sliced
175 g (6 oz) Chinese leaves, trimmed and thinly sliced
1 red pepper, cored, seeded and thinly sliced
2 tbsp tamari sauce

1. Place the peanuts on a baking dish in a pre-heated oven 190°C/375°F/gas mark 5 until they are lightly roasted.
2. Heat the oil in a wok or heavy frying pan and stir fry the tempeh on both sides until lightly browned.
3. Slice the orange segments crossways into triangles. Add the cayenne, cumin, spring onions, garlic and Chinese leaves and toss in the oil for 1 minute.
4. Add the roasted peanuts and red pepper, mix and fry again for 1 minute.
5. Lastly add the orange triangles and tamari sauce and stir-fry until all the tempeh and vegetables are coated and the oranges are heated through. Serve immediately.

SERVES 4

TOFU RISOTTO

225 g (8 oz) brown rice
1 tbsp soya oil
225 g (8 oz) tofu cut into 2.5 cm (1-inch) cubes
1 medium onion
1 clove garlic
1 red pepper, seeded and sliced
1 green pepper, seeded and sliced
50 g (2 oz) green beans
100 g (4 oz) carrots, cut into matchsticks

100 g (4 oz) courgettes, thinly sliced
100 g (4 oz) broccoli, broken into florets and stalk sliced
1 small orange, broken into segments and skin removed
1 tbsp flaked almonds
1 tbsp fresh chopped parsley

1. Cook the rice as directed on the packet and put to one side.
2. Heat the oil in a large frying pan and add the tofu, onion, garlic and red and green peppers and gently fry for 2–3 minutes.
3. Steam the beans, carrots, courgettes and broccoli over a pan of boiling water for 5 minutes (alternatively leave out the steaming if you like your vegetables crunchy), add to the other ingredients in the frying pan.
4. Add the sautéed tofu, orange, flaked almonds, parsley and rice and heat thoroughly. Serve immediately.

SERVES 4

TOFU 'MEAT' BALLS

1 onion
100 g (4 oz) fresh parsley
275 g (10 oz) tofu
50 g (2 oz) fresh breadcrumbs
1 egg
1 tsp dried basil
1 tsp dried oregano
1 garlic clove

1 tsp ground nutmeg
black pepper
50 g (2 oz) fresh Parmesan cheese,
  grated
150 g (5 oz) tomato purée
50 g (2 oz) soya flour

1. Pre-heat the oven to 180°C/350°F/gas mark 4.
2. Place the onion and parsley in a food processor and process until smooth.
3. Add the tofu, breadcrumbs, egg, herbs, garlic, pepper, cheese and 3 tablespoons of the tomato purée. Process until all the ingredients are combined.
4. Form into 16 balls the size of a walnut, then dust each with the soya flour.
5. Grease a baking tray and cook for 35 minutes.
6. Transfer the 'meat' balls to a large saucepan and add the remaining tomato purée, cover and simmer for 10 minutes or until the sauce is hot.
7. Serve with rice or potatoes and vegetables.

SERVES 4

SESAME TOFU

50 ml (2 fl oz) tamari sauce
2 tbsp water
1 tbsp rice vinegar
1 tsp brown sugar
1 tsp sesame oil

1 spring onion, finely chopped
1 tsp fresh root ginger, finely
  chopped
275 g (10 oz) tofu
1 tbsp sesame seeds

1. Mix the tamari sauce, water, vinegar, sugar, sesame oil, spring onion and ginger in a bowl.
2. Cut the tofu into 2.5 cm (1-inch) cubes and place in the marinade. Refrigerate for at least 1 hour.
3. Pre-heat the oven to 220°C/450°F/gas mark 8.
4. In a dry frying pan, roast the sesame seeds until lightly browned. Press the seeds into the tofu and bake in the oven for 10 minutes or until lightly browned.
5. Serve with a salad for lunch or with rice or noodles and stir-fried mixed vegetables for a more substantial meal.

SERVES 2

'POLENTA' PIE

450 g (1 lb) cornmeal
900 ml (1 1/2 pints) So Good soya
    milk
50 g (2 oz) soya margarine

For the filling
100 g (4 oz) textured vegetable
    protein (TVP)

450 g (1 lb) mixed vegetables
    (courgettes, red and green
    pepper, aubergine etc.)
1 tsp ground coriander
1 tsp dried thyme
black pepper
300 ml (1/2 pint) vegetable stock

1. Pre-heat the oven to 180°C/350°F/gas mark 4 and grease a medium-sized oven dish.
2. Measure the cornmeal into a bowl with 300 ml (1/2 pint) of the So Good and stir to make a smooth paste. Heat the rest of the So Good in a saucepan and, when it has come to the boil, add the margarine and the cornmeal paste. Stir often over the next 5–10 minutes while the mixture thickens to make a slightly stiff dough.
3. Remove the mixture from the heat and press about two-thirds of the cornmeal dough into the greased oven dish. A wet spoon will enable you to press the hot dough into place more easily.
4. Meanwhile, prepare the filling for the pie. Mix the TVP with the vegetables and other ingredients and turn into the polenta-lined dish.
5. Roll out the remaining cornmeal dough on a floured surface and place over the filling. Press and trim the edges. Brush the top of the pie with a little oil if you like a crispy texture. Serve hot with rice and vegetables.

SERVES 4–6

SALADS

BROWN RICE AND WATERCRESS SALAD

50 g (2 oz) brown rice, cooked
1 bunch of watercress, washed and
    chopped
100 g (4 oz) tinned or frozen
    sweetcorn, cooked and drained

1 green pepper, de-seeded and
    chopped
black pepper, to taste

Mix all the ingredients together and season with black pepper.

SERVES 4

TROPICAL RICE SALAD

175 g (6 oz) long-grain rice
1/2 tsp ground turmeric
450 ml (3/4 pint) vegetable stock
2 ripe bananas
2 tbsp lemon juice

1/2 pineapple, peeled, cored and
  chopped
100 g (4 oz) organic sultanas
1/2 cucumber, cubed

1. Put the rice, turmeric and vegetable stock in a saucepan and bring to the boil. Reduce the heat and simmer for 10–15 minutes. Drain thoroughly and allow to cool.
2. Peel and slice the bananas and toss in the lemon juice.
3. Mix the rice, banana, pineapple, sultanas and cucumber together and put in a salad bowl.

SERVES 4–6

APPLE AND NUT SALAD

4 red apples, wiped
lemon juice, to coat
1/2 cucumber, thickly sliced

6 celery sticks, chopped
1 bunch of spring onions, sliced
75 g (3 oz) natural peanuts

1. Core and roughly chop the apples and dip them in the lemon juice to prevent discolouration. Cut the cucumber slices into quarters.
2. Mix all the ingredients together and toss in the dressing of your choice. See Sauces and Dressings on page 223.

SERVES 4

ENDIVE, FRUIT AND NUT SALAD

2 heads curly endive lettuce
3 oranges
25 g (1 oz) flaked almonds
25 g (1 oz) walnuts, chopped

2 apples, washed, cored and sliced
  into small segments
75 g (3 oz) seedless white grapes
1 tbsp lemon juice

1. Pull the endive apart, wash and dry it thoroughly. Tear the leaves into pieces and place in a salad bowl.
2. Grate the rind of one orange into a bowl. Remove the peel and pith from all the oranges, break them into segments and place in a separate bowl.
3. Mix together the almonds, walnuts, apple, grapes and lemon juice and add to the oranges. Mix well.
4. Place the fruit and nut mixture in the bowl on top of the endive. Chill before serving with a dressing of your choice.

SERVES 4 (main course); 8 (starter/side dish)

SEAFOOD SALAD

350 g (12 oz) cod fillet
1/2 white cabbage, trimmed
225 g (8 oz) peeled prawns
100 g (4 oz) cooked mussels,
    shelled

1 onion, grated
100 g (4 oz) carrots, grated
1 tsp chopped fresh dill

1. Steam the cod until tender, then remove the skin and flake the fish. Leave to cool.
2. Shred the cabbage finely, then rinse and drain well. Pat dry with a clean cloth or kitchen paper.
3. Mix together the cod, cabbage, prawns, mussels, onion, carrots and dill.
4. Toss the salad with the dressing of your choice.

SERVES 4

COLESLAW

1 medium white cabbage, cored and
    finely shredded
5 medium carrots, coarsely grated
1 medium onion, finely chopped

50 g (2 oz) organic raisins
4 tbsp natural soya yogurt
4 tbsp soya mayonnaise
black pepper, to taste

1. Mix the cabbage, carrots, onion and raisins in a large bowl.
2. Add the soya mayonnaise and yogurt and black pepper, and toss gently to coat all the ingredients.

SERVES 6

ORANGE AND AVOCADO SALAD

2 avocados (skins and stones
    removed)
2 oranges (peeled and chopped)
1 spring onion, finely chopped
2 tbsp lemon juice

2 tbsp orange juice
2 tsp linseed (flaxseed) oil
1/4 tsp chopped fresh ginger
lettuce leaves

Cut the avocados into slices lengthways. Mix with the orange pieces and spring onion. Mix together the lemon juice, orange juice, oil and ginger and pour over the salad. Serve on the lettuce leaves.

SERVES 4

SWEET POTATO SALAD

450 g (1 lb) orange fleshed sweet
   potatoes
1 tbsp soya oil
3 tbsp lemon juice
1–2 cloves garlic, crushed

1 tbsp chopped parsley
1 tbsp chopped basil
1 tbsp chopped chives
1 tbsp chopped spring onion

Steam the sweet potatoes until tender but not mushy. Dice and place in a bowl. Add the remaining ingredients and combine.

SERVES 6

APPLE, CELERY AND BEETROOT SALAD

1 eating apple, sliced (leave skin
   on)
1 large cooked beetroot, cubed

1 tbsp French dressing
1 stick celery, diced
1 tbsp chopped walnuts

Combine all the ingredients and mix well.

SERVES 4

AVOCADO, SMOKED TOFU AND PINEAPPLE SALAD

1 large avocado, peeled and diced
175 g (6 oz) diced smoked tofu

1 cup chopped pineapple

Combine the ingredients and serve with a dressing if wished.

SERVES 4

HAZELNUT AND RICE SALAD

175 g (6 oz) cooked brown rice
1/2 tsp ground cinnamon
2 tbsp toasted sesame seeds
6 chopped dried organic apricots

2 tbsp French dressing
2 tbsp organic raisins
2 tbsp toasted, chopped hazelnuts
1 tsp grated ginger

Combine all the ingredients and mix well.

SERVES 4

APPLE, CARROT AND GINGER SALAD

1 grated apple
1 large carrot

1 tbsp grated ginger
1 tbsp French dressing

Combine the ingredients and mix well.

SERVES 4

CARROT AND RAISIN SALAD

275 g (10 oz) grated carrot
50 g (2 oz) desiccated coconut

2 tbsp chopped organic raisins
juice of 1/2 orange

Mix all the ingredients together.

SERVES 4

SAUCES AND DRESSINGS

ORANGE SAUCE

100 ml (4 fl oz) white wine vinegar
1 tbsp sugar
225 ml (8 fl oz) fresh orange juice,
  strained

1 tsp cornflour
1 tbsp water

1. Put the vinegar and sugar in a saucepan and stir over a medium heat until the sugar has dissolved. Boil rapidly until the mixture turns a light golden brown.
2. Stir the orange juice into the saucepan and bring back to the boil. Reduce the heat and simmer until the liquid has reduced by about half.
3. Blend the cornflour with the water and add to the saucepan. Cook over a low heat, stirring constantly, until the mixture thickens.

SERVES 4

MUSTARD DRESSING

100 ml (4 fl oz) freshly squeezed
   lemon juice
1 tbsp French whole-grain mustard

1 tbsp chopped fresh parsley
3 tbsp water

Whisk all the ingredients together until well combined. Cover and chill before serving.

ORANGE CHILLI DRESSING

2 tbsp tamari sauce
3 tbsp orange juice
1 small fresh green chilli, de-seeded
   and chopped

1 garlic clove, crushed

Whisk all the ingredients together until well combined. Cover and chill before serving.

TAMARI AND GINGER DRESSING

150 ml (1/4 pint) soya oil
50 ml (2 fl oz) rice wine vinegar
1 tbsp tamari sauce

25 g (1 oz) fresh ginger, grated
3 garlic cloves, crushed

Blend the ingredients thoroughly.

TAHINI AND LEMON DRESSING

275 ml (10 fl oz) hot water
150 g (5 oz) tahini
juice of 1 lemon
100 ml (4 fl oz) olive oil

275 ml (10 fl oz) natural soya
   yogurt
3 garlic cloves, crushed
black pepper

1. Stir the hot water into the tahini to create a thick paste – allow to cool.
2. Blend the lemon juice and olive oil with the tahini paste until smooth.
3. Fold the soya yogurt into the mixture with the garlic. Season to taste.

ALMOND CHILLI DRESSING

50 ml (2 fl oz) soya oil
1 medium onion, thinly sliced
1/2 tsp chilli
1 dsp honey
1 tsp tamari
1 tbsp tomato purée

2–3 tbsp almond butter
3 garlic cloves, crushed
300 ml (1/2 pint) cold water
300 ml (1/2 pint) So Good soya
    milk
black pepper

1. Heat the oil gently and stir in the onion, chilli, honey and tamari. Cook until the onion is soft.
2. Stir in the tomato purée, almond butter and garlic and bring to the boil, stirring continuously.
3. Pour the water and So Good over the almond mixture and bring back to the boil, stirring regularly until it is smooth and not too thick. Season to taste and allow to cool.

AVOCADO DRESSING

1 large avocado
1 large tomato
1 spring onion, chopped

2 tsp chopped fresh dill
1 tsp chopped fresh oregano

Blend the ingredients and serve over vegetables or cooked rice.

TOFU DRESSING

100 g (4 oz) tofu, mashed
2 tbsp lemon juice
3 tbsp tahini
1 tsp tamari sauce

1 tbsp finely chopped spring onion
1 tbsp finely chopped chives
1 tbsp finely chopped parsley

Blend the tofu, lemon juice, tahini and tamari. Stir in the spring onion, chives and parsley.

TAHINI MAYONNAISE

4 tbsp tahini

4 tbsp lemon juice

2 tsp honey

2–3 tsp tamari sauce

2 tsp cider vinegar

1/4 tsp ground mustard

Stir the ingredients until thoroughly blended – it should have quite a thick consistency.

SPICY PEANUT SAUCE

3 garlic cloves, finely chopped

1 large onion, finely chopped

1 tbsp fresh ginger, grated

1–2 fresh chillies, finely chopped

100 g (4 oz) chopped peanuts

150 ml (1/4 pint) peanut butter

600 ml (1 pint) vegetable stock

1 tsp chilli powder

1 tbsp tamari sauce

juice of 1 lemon

1. Heat the oil in a saucepan and slowly sweat the garlic and onion until clear and tender, about 15 minutes. Add the ginger and the chillies and stir for 2 minutes.
2. Add the chopped peanuts and stir for 5 minutes. Stir the peanut butter into the sautéed ingredients and when it has melted a little, add half the stock. Keep stirring as you bring the sauce to a low boil.
3. The sauce will thicken, and at this stage, add the chilli powder and tamari sauce. Add more stock to make a smooth, pourable sauce but one that is not too runny.
4. Add the lemon juice when the sauce is ready, but keep it over the heat for a further 2–3 minutes while you stir the juice in. Remove from the heat and serve hot over steamed vegetables or meat.

MAKES 600 ml (1 pint)

DESSERTS

APRICOT SQUARES

100 g (4 oz) organic dried apricots
150 ml (1/4 pint) water
50 g (2 oz) potato flour
50 g (2 oz) soya flour
1 1/2 tsp baking powder

100 g (4 oz) porridge oats
50 g (2 oz) unrefined sugar
100 g (4 oz) soya margarine
2 tbsp honey

1. Place the apricots in a pan with the water and bring to the boil. Simmer gently, stirring occasionally, until all the water has been absorbed and the apricots are tender. Beat mixture until smooth.
2. Sieve the flour and baking powder into a bowl and stir in the oats and sugar. Rub in the margarine until the mixture begins to stick together. Warm the honey so it is slightly runny and mix into the cake mixture.
3. Press half the cake mixture into the base of an 18 cm (7-inch) square tin. Spread the apricots over this and then top with the remaining mixture. Spread evenly.
4. Bake at 190°C/375°F/gas mark 5 for 35–40 minutes, until the cake is golden brown. Leave to become quite cold in the tin, cut into squares and remove.

PARKIN

225 g (8 oz) barley flour
1 tsp baking powder
2 tsp ground ginger
100 g (4 oz) soya margarine
225 g (8 oz) medium oatmeal

100 g (4 oz) unrefined sugar
225 g (8 oz) molasses
75 ml (3 fl oz) pure apple juice
75 ml (3 fl oz) water

1. Sieve the barley flour, baking powder and ginger into a bowl. Rub in the margarine, then stir in the oatmeal and sugar.
2. Warm the molasses, then pour with the apple juice and water into the centre of the dry ingredients. Beat lightly until thoroughly blended.
3. Turn the mixture into a greased 23 cm (9-inch) square tin. Bake at 180°C/350°F/gas mark 4 for 40–50 minutes.
4. Leave to cool in the tin for 10 minutes before transferring to a wire rack.

This cake is moist so it keeps well – it improves after about 1 week.

RHUBARB AND GINGER WHIP

675 g (1 1/2 lb) rhubarb
2 tbsp clear honey
225 g (8 oz) silken tofu

1 piece stem or crystallised ginger
25 g (1 oz) flaked almonds

1. Trim the rhubarb, removing any coarse stringy pieces. Cut into 1 cm (1/2-inch) lengths and cook gently with a little water until soft.
2. Sweeten with honey. Put the tofu into a blender, add the rhubarb mixture and blend.
3. Stir in the finely chopped ginger and divide between 4 dishes. Sprinkle flaked almonds over the top.

SERVES 4

PRUNE AND TOFU DESSERT

100 g (4 oz) organic prunes
225 g (8 oz) silken tofu

2 tbsp natural maple syrup or clear honey

1. Soak the prunes overnight. Drain and place in a saucepan with sufficient fresh water to cover. Simmer for 10–15 minutes until really tender.
2. Drain again (reserving the liquor) and place in a liquidiser with the tofu and syrup or honey, and blend thoroughly.
3. Add just enough cooking liquor to make a thick but soft purée and blend. Pour into 4 sundae glasses and chill until ready to serve.

SERVES 4

GINGER FRUIT SALAD

juice of 2 oranges
3 tbsp juice from stem ginger jar
25 g (1 oz) unrefined soft brown sugar
2 oranges

1 ogen melon
3 dessert apples
2 pieces of preserved stem ginger, finely chopped
fresh mint leaves, to decorate

1. Put the orange juice in a saucepan with the stem ginger juice and sugar. Heat gently until the sugar has dissolved. Bring to the boil and boil for about 5 minutes or until syrupy. Remove from the heat and leave to cool.

2. Peel the oranges, removing the pith, and slice into thick rings. Cut the rings into quarters, removing any pips.
3. Cut the melon in half, remove the seeds and scoop out the flesh, using a melon baller if possible.
4. Peel and core the apples, then chop roughly.
5. Put all the fruit into a serving bowl, or into the empty melon halves, with the ginger and sugar syrup. Stir well, cover and chill for 1–2 hours. Decorate with mint.

SERVES 4–6

CINNAMON RHUBARB

300 g (11 oz) rhubarb
4 tbsp water
pinch ground cinnamon

50 g (2 oz) unrefined soft brown sugar

1. Wash, trim and chop the rhubarb.
2. Put the rhubarb in a saucepan with the water, cinnamon and sugar and stew until the rhubarb is tender.
3. Spoon into dishes and serve with soya yogurt or custard.

SERVES 4

BANANA AND TOFU CREAM

200 g (7 oz) firm tofu
200 g (7 oz) bananas, peeled
75 g (3 oz) ground almonds

1 pinch of cinnamon
2 tsp almond flakes

1. Blend or process the tofu and banana together. To obtain a creamy texture, the mixture may need to be put through a sieve.
2. Add the ground almonds and mix well.
3. Spoon into 4 bowls and sprinkle with the cinnamon and a few almond flakes.

SERVES 4

APPLE AND TOFU CHEESECAKE

1 quantity of pastry (see Pastry on
   page 245)

Filling
450 g (1 lb) eating apples, chopped
100 ml (4 fl oz) water
200 g (7 oz) firm tofu

1 egg white, whisked
2 tbsp freshly squeezed lemon
   juice
1 tsp vanilla essence
1 tsp cinnamon
25 g (1 oz) ground almonds
25 g (1 oz) brown rice flakes

1. Bake the pastry blind in a 23 cm (9-inch) baking tin for 10 minutes
   in a pre-heated oven 180°C/350°F/gas mark 4.
2. Combine the apple with the water and purée in a blender or food
   processor. Add the tofu and continue to blend until a thick paste is
   formed.
3. Fold in the whisked egg white, lemon juice, vanilla essence, cinnamon and ground almonds.
4. Pour the mixture into the part-baked pastry case and sprinkle with
   the brown rice flakes.
5. Return to the oven at the same temperature for 30 minutes.
6. Serve chilled.

MAKES 12 SLICES

RHUBARB FOOL WITH TOFU LEMON CREAM

4 medium cooking apples
6 medium rhubarb stalks
honey to taste
cinnamon
pecan nuts

Tofu lemon cream
400 g (14 oz) silken tofu
50 ml (2 fl oz) lemon juice
grated rind of 2 lemons
pure maple syrup to taste

1. Slice the apples finely and chop the rhubarb into small chunks.
   Cook with a little water and honey and refrigerate until cold.
2. Blend the tofu, lemon juice, rind and maple syrup until smooth.
3. Layer the rhubarb mixture and tofu cream in tall glasses. Finish with
   a layer of the cream and top with cinnamon and crumbled pecan
   nuts. Serve well chilled.

SERVES 4

BAKED BANANA AND RICE PUDDING

1 cup uncooked brown rice
1 cup mashed banana
750 ml (11/4 pints) So Good soya
  milk, unsweetened or sweetened

1 tsp pure vanilla essence
rind of 1 lemon
1 tsp nutmeg

1. Place all the ingredients in a casserole dish, except the nutmeg. Stir well. Sprinkle nutmeg over the top, using a tea strainer to shake evenly.
2. Bake for 1^{1}/$_{2}$–2 hours at 180°C/350°F/gas mark 4. Serve on its own, or with stewed fruit.

SERVES 4

FRUIT AND NUT COMPOTE

This is a delicious variation on a traditional compote – the addition of the nuts and tangy citrus sauce makes a wonderful difference! It makes a lovely breakfast.

juice and rind of 1 orange
juice and rind of 1 lemon
150 ml (1/4 pint) pure apple juice
100 g (4 oz) organic dried apricots
100 g (4 oz) dried apple rings
100 g (4 oz) organic sultanas
100 g (4 oz) organic raisins

100 g (4 oz) organic prunes
50 g (2 oz) pecan nuts, chopped
50 g (2 oz) almonds
50 g (2 oz) hazelnuts
2 tbsp sunflower seeds
2 tbsp golden linseeds

1. Combine all the ingredients and leave to soak overnight. The fruit should be plump and juicy.
2. Serve chilled with plenty of natural bio or soya yogurt.

SERVES 4

RASPBERRY AND TOFU BRÛLÉE

275 g (10 oz) packet silken tofu
2 tbsp clear honey

200 g (7 oz) raspberries, frozen
3 tbsp unrefined soft brown sugar

1. Place the tofu, honey and raspberries in a food processor or liquidiser, and blend until smooth.
2. Divide the mixture between 4 ramekin dishes.
3. Sprinkle the sugar over each dish and place under a hot grill until golden and the sugar forms a hard layer.

SERVES 4

RHUBARB CRUMBLE

900 g (2 lb) rhubarb, washed and
  trimmed
175 g (6 oz) unrefined brown sugar
225 g (8 oz) rolled oats

50 g (2 oz) rice flour
50 g (2 oz) soya flour
1 tsp ground cinnamon
75 g (3 oz) soya margarine

1. Mix the rhubarb with 75 g (3 oz) of the sugar and turn into a 23 x 33 cm (9 x 13-inch) baking dish. Leave the fruit to stand for 10–15 minutes then stir and distribute evenly in the dish.
2. Mix the oats, flours, remaining sugar and cinnamon together and work in the margarine to make a crumbly texture.
3. Spread this mixture over the rhubarb and lightly press into place. Bake for 20 minutes, in a pre-heated oven at 180°C/350°F/gas mark 4 until the topping is golden. Serve hot with Soya Dream or soya yogurt.

SERVES 4

BANANA LEMON WHIP

2 small bananas
175 g (6 oz) silken tofu
juice of 1/2 lemon

1 tbsp honey
1/2 tsp tahini

Combine all the ingredients in a blender and purée until smooth. Serve immediately in dishes or as a topping for pancakes, crêpes or waffles.

SERVES 2

NUT CRUNCH WITH TOFU WHIPPED CREAM

2 bananas, cut into rounds
50 g (2 oz) chopped almonds
50 g (2 oz) chopped walnuts
50 g (2 oz) sunflower seeds
50 g (2 oz) organic raisins
50 g (2 oz) chopped organic pitted
   dates

50 g (2 oz) shredded coconut
350 g (12 oz) silken tofu
2 tbsp clear honey
1/2 tsp natural vanilla essence

1. Combine the first seven ingredients together in a large bowl; mix well and set aside.
2. Purée the tofu, honey and vanilla until smooth.
3. Serve the fruit and nut mixture with the tofu cream.

SERVES 6

TOFU-STRAWBERRY DESSERT

700 g (24 oz) tofu, chilled and
   mashed
2 tbsp honey
2 tsp natural vanilla essence

15 strawberries, cut vertically into
   halves
50 g (2 oz) sliced almonds, toasted

1. Combine the tofu, honey and vanilla in a large bowl and mix well with a fork.
2. Place the strawberries on top of the tofu mixture and sprinkle with almonds.

SERVES 6

TOFU ORANGE ALMOND DESSERT

150 ml (1/4 pint) fresh unsweetened
   orange juice
2 tbsp clear honey
1 1/2 tsp grated orange rind
1/4 tsp almond essence

350 g (12 oz) tofu, cut into 1 cm
   (1/2-inch) cubes
100 g (4 oz) tangerine segments
3 tbsp sliced almonds, toasted

1. Combine the orange juice and honey in a small bowl and simmer uncovered until reduced and slightly thickened.
2. Stir in the orange rind and almond essence, then combine with the tofu and tangerines in a bowl. Cover and chill for at least 2 hours.
3. Serve in small bowls decorated with the toasted almonds.

SERVES 3

'CRÈME CARAMEL'

50 g (2 oz) unrefined sugar
2 tbsp cold water
1 tbsp boiling water
3 large eggs

300 ml (1/2 pint) So Good soya milk
25 g (1 oz) unrefined caster sugar
1/2 tsp vanilla essence
150 ml (1/4 pint) Soya Dream

1. Put the sugar and cold water into a small saucepan and heat gently until the sugar dissolves. Bring to the boil, then boil more briskly – without stirring – until the syrup turns a deep golden colour.
2. Remove from the heat and stir in the boiling water. Pour into a greased 600 ml (1 pint) heatproof dish. Tilt the dish so the base is completely covered with caramel.
3. Beat the eggs with the So Good, add the caster sugar and vanilla and mix well.
4. Strain the mixture into the dish and stand it in a roasting tin containing enough cold water to come halfway up the sides of the dish.
5. Place in a pre-heated oven at 160°C/325°F/gas mark 3 for 3/4 to 1 hour. Remove from the oven and cool.
6. Turn out on to a serving dish and chill before serving. Serve with Soya Dream.

SERVES 4

STUFFED DATES

450 g (1 lb) fresh dates
275 g (10 oz) plain firm tofu
100 g (4 oz) ground almonds

225 g (8 oz) Soya Dream
1 tsp ground cinnamon
100 g (4 oz) whole almonds

1. Slice the dates in half and remove the stones. Leave each date open.
2. Mash the tofu in a bowl and blend the ground almonds into it. Add the Soya Dream, a little at a time, and stir well after each addition. Stir in the cinnamon.
3. Spoon the mixture into the dates and decorate with a whole almond. Chill before serving.

SERVES 4

ELDERFLOWER SORBET

225 g (8 oz) unrefined granulated   2 lemons
    sugar   2 good elderflower heads
600 ml (1 pint) water

1. Place the sugar and water in a saucepan. Heat gently, stirring well until the sugar has dissolved.
2. Add thinly pared lemon rind and boil for 5 minutes. Remove from the heat, add the elderflower heads and squeezed lemon juice. Leave to cool, then strain and freeze, stirring all the edges to the middle as they harden.
3. When it has all set fairly hard beat well until the mixture is soft and light. Re-freeze. Remove and put in the fridge 40 minutes before required.

SERVES 4

CAKES AND BISCUITS

ALMOND BISCUITS

100 g (4 oz) soya margarine   50 g (2 oz) rice flour
100 g (4 oz) unrefined brown sugar   1 egg
100 g (4 oz) ground almonds   50 g (2 oz) chopped almonds
50 g (2 oz) cornflour

1. Cream the margarine and sugar together, then work in the ground almonds and flour.
2. Separate the egg yolk and keep a little of the white.
3. Beat the rest of the egg and add a little at a time to the mixture, working it in until a firm dough is produced.
4. Roll out 3 mm (1/8 inch) thick and cut into rounds or shapes.
5. Brush the dough with the egg white and decorate with the chopped almonds.
6. Bake in a pre-heated oven, 180°C/350°F/gas mark 4 for 10–12 minutes or until they are golden brown.
7. Cool on a wire tray and store in an airtight container.

MAKES 48 SMALL BISCUITS

GINGER SNAPS

25 g (1 oz) potato flour   25 g (1 oz) cornflour
25 g (1 oz) rice flour   75 g (3 oz) soya flour

1/2 tsp bicarbonate of soda
1/2 tsp cream of tartar
2 tsp ground ginger
100 g (4 oz) unrefined sugar

50 g (2 oz) soya margarine
40 g (1 1/2 oz) golden syrup
1 egg, beaten

1. Sift all the dry ingredients together.
2. Melt the margarine and the syrup together and allow these to cool slightly before adding to the dry mixture.
3. Add the egg to the mixture, which now should form a firm dough.
4. Shape the dough into walnut-sized balls and place them well apart on a greased tray.
5. Bake in a pre-heated oven, 190°C/375°F/gas mark 5 for 15–20 minutes or until they are brown.

MAKES 24

CHEWY FRUIT BARS

100 g (4 oz) dried organic apricots
100 ml (4 fl oz) orange juice
1 tsp grated orange rind
50 g (2 oz) almonds, chopped
50 g (2 oz) desiccated coconut

50 g (2 oz) puffed rice cereal
100 g (4 oz) ground almonds
50 g (2 oz) dried fruit, e.g. raisins, apple, peach
extra desiccated coconut

1. Cut the apricots into small pieces and simmer in the orange juice and rind for approximately 5 minutes or until soft.
2. Toast the chopped almonds in the oven or under the grill. Toast the desiccated coconut in the same way but make sure that it does not burn.
3. Put the puffed rice, coconut, ground almonds and apricot mixture in a mixer and process until well mixed. You will need to stop the machine and scrape the mixture from the sides of the bowl once or twice as the mixture is quite sticky.
4. Turn the mixture out into a bowl and add the chopped toasted nuts and chopped dried fruit. Mix by hand until the mixture forms a large ball.
5. Line a baking tray with foil or greaseproof paper and sprinkle with desiccated coconut. Spread the mixture out, levelling the surface, and sprinkle with more coconut. Press down well, cut into 12 or 16 pieces then leave to dry out, preferably overnight, before storing in an airtight container. Use within 1 week.

MAKES 12–16

GINGER AND ORANGE CAKE

100 g (4 oz) potato flour
50 g (2 oz) ground almonds
50 g (2 oz) banana
1 tsp orange rind
1 tsp ground ginger
1 egg

50 g (2 oz) soya flour
1 tbsp soya oil
juice of 1 orange made up to
    150 ml (1/4 pint) with water
2 tsp baking powder
75 g (3 oz) organic sultanas

1. If a food processor is available, place all the ingredients except the sultanas in the goblet and process until smooth and well mixed. Alternatively, beat the egg in a bowl and add the remaining ingredients, beating well with a wooden spoon.
2. Add and mix in the sultanas.
3. Place the mixture in a 450 g (1 lb) greased loaf tin and bake in the centre of the oven at 200°C/400°F/gas mark 6 for approximately 30 minutes or until golden brown and firm to the touch.
4. Turn out of the tin and cool on a wire tray. Keep covered in a container in the fridge and eat within 3 days.

ALMOND LOAF

3 egg whites
pinch of cream of tartar
75 g (3 oz) clear honey
1 tsp almond essence

150 g (5 oz) rice flour
50 g (2 oz) blanched almonds,
    halved

1. Beat the egg whites with the cream of tartar. Gradually fold in the honey and almond essence until the mixture is of a meringue consistency, forming thick peaks.
2. Fold in the flour and almonds and spoon into a greased 450 g (1 lb) loaf tin. Bake in a pre-heated oven at 180°C/350°F/gas mark 4 for 30–40 minutes.

SESAME SQUARES

175 g (6 oz) sesame seeds
75 g (3 oz) desiccated coconut
50 g (2 oz) almond butter
100 g (4 oz) clear honey
1/2 tsp vanilla essence
100 g (4 oz) chopped mixed nuts
225 g (8 oz) oats
100 g (4 oz) organic raisins, chopped

1. Mix all the ingredients together thoroughly. Press into a greased 18 cm (7-inch) square cake tin.
2. Bake in a pre-heated oven at 180°C/350°F/gas mark 4 for about 30 minutes until lightly browned. When cold cut into squares.

MAKES 12

APRICOT COCONUT BALLS

225 g (8 oz) dried organic apricots, soaked in boiling water until soft
1 tsp lemon juice
2 tbsp orange juice
225 g (8 oz) desiccated coconut
2 tsp orange rind

1. Drain the water from the apricots and chop finely. Mix with the remaining ingredients.
2. Roll into small balls, then roll in the coconut. Chill until firm.

CHOCOLATE FRUIT SLICE

175 g (6 oz) soya chocolate
175 g (6 oz) mixed dried fruit
50 g (2 oz) natural dried cherries
50 g (2 oz) chopped almonds
50 g (2 oz) shredded coconut
50 g (2 oz) unrefined sugar
25 g (1 oz) soya margarine
1 egg, beaten

1. Melt the soya chocolate and spread it evenly in the base of a foil-lined shallow 20 x 15 cm (8 x 6-inch) tin. Leave this in the fridge to cool until set.
2. Mix all the other ingredients together and spread over the solid chocolate in the tin.
3. Bake in a pre-heated oven, 180°C/350°F/gas mark 4 for 20–25 minutes until the top is golden brown.
4. When the tin is cool, place in the fridge for at least 1 hour until cold. Cut into fingers and turn out of the tin.

MAKES 12 SLICES

NUTTY FLAPJACKS

150 g (5 oz) soya margarine
50 g (4 oz) unrefined soft brown
  sugar
1 tbsp brown rice syrup*
1 tbsp clear honey

225 g (8 oz) oats
50 g (2 oz) pecan nuts, chopped
50 g (2 oz) almonds, chopped
2 tbsp golden linseeds

1. Melt the margarine, sugar, syrup and honey over a moderate heat.
2. Stir the oats, nuts and linseeds into the syrup mixture and stir until well combined.
3. Turn out into a 20 cm (8-inch) square tin and bake in a pre-heated oven at 180°C/350°F/gas mark 4 for 20 minutes, or until lightly golden.

MAKES 12

*a golden syrup substitute available from healthfood shops

ALMOND AND CINNAMON FLAPJACKS

150 g (5 oz) soya margarine
50 g (4 oz) unrefined soft brown
  sugar
1 tbsp brown rice syrup*
1 tbsp clear honey

175 g (6 oz) oats
50 g (2 oz) ground almonds
50 g (2 oz) almonds, chopped
1 tsp ground cinnamon

1. Melt the margarine, sugar, syrup and honey over a moderate heat.
2. Stir the oats, ground almonds, chopped almonds and the cinnamon into the syrup mixture and stir until well combined.
3. Turn out into a 20 cm (8-inch) square tin and bake in a pre-heated oven at 180°C/350°F/gas mark 4 for 20 minutes, or until lightly golden.

MAKES 12

*a golden syrup substitute available from healthfood shops

COCONUT BROWNIES

50 g (2 oz) soya chocolate
75 g (3 oz) soya margarine
2 eggs
175 g (6 oz) unrefined brown sugar
75 g (3 oz) soya flour
1/2 tsp wheat-free baking powder

75 g (3 oz) desiccated coconut

Topping
25 g (1 oz) soya margarine
2 tbsp unrefined soft brown sugar
100 g (4 oz) desiccated coconut

1. Melt the soya chocolate and margarine over a gentle heat. Set aside to cool. Beat the eggs until fluffy and gradually add the sugar and beat until well blended.
2. Add the melted chocolate mixture, flour, baking powder and coconut. Beat well and spread in a greased 20 cm (8-inch) square tin.
3. To make the topping: melt the margarine and stir in the sugar and coconut. Spread evenly over the cake batter and bake for 30 minutes at 180°C/350°F/gas mark
4. Cool in the tin and cut into 12 squares. Transfer to a wire rack until completely cold.

MAKES 12

CHERRY GINGER CAKE

150 g (5 oz) crystallised ginger
75 g (3 oz) natural glacé cherries
150 g (5 oz) soya margarine
150 g (5 oz) unrefined brown sugar
3 medium size eggs
50 g (2 oz) rice flour

50 g (2 oz) potato flour
50 g (2 oz) soya flour
50 g (2 oz) ground almonds
few drops of vanilla essence
1 tbsp So Good soya milk

1. Cut the ginger into small pieces, and halve the cherries, rinse them in water then roll them in flour.
2. Cream the soya margarine and sugar until pale and fluffy, then beat eggs and add to the creamed mixture. Add the sifted flour and ground almonds and beat well until smooth. Add the vanilla essence and So Good and stir thoroughly.
3. Turn into a greased 900 g (2 lb) loaf tin and bake at 180°C/350°F/gas mark 4 for 50 minutes, then reduce to 160°C/325°F/gas mark 3 for a further 25–30 minutes, until golden brown.

SERVES 12

BREADS AND SCONES

HONEY LOAF

100 g (4 oz) potato flour
100 g (4 oz) rice flour
100 g (4 oz) soya flour
1 tsp bicarbonate of soda
1/2 tsp cream of tartar
1/4 tsp tartaric acid
3 tsp mixed spice

50 g (2 oz) candied peel, chopped finely
100 g (4 oz) unrefined sugar
175 g (6 oz) clear honey
150 ml (1/4 pint) So Good soya milk

1. Mix all the flours together with the raising agents.
2. Add the remaining ingredients, except the So Good.
3. Add the So Good and mix until the mixture will flow slowly.
4. Pour the mixture into a greased 900 g (2 lb) loaf tin.
5. Bake in a pre-heated oven, 200°C/400°F/gas mark 6, for 30 minutes and then reduce the temperature to 150°C/300°F/gas mark 2 until cooked through. Check by using a skewer through the middle. The loaf is not cooked until the skewer comes out clean.
6. Allow to stand for 10 minutes before turning out on to a wire tray to cool thoroughly.

MAKES ONE 675 g (1^1/$_2$lb) LOAF

SAVOURY CRACKERS

150 g (5 oz) rice flour
75 g (3 oz) ground almonds
1 tbsp finely chopped onion

2 tsp tamari sauce
100 ml (4 fl oz) water
sesame seeds

1. Mix together the flour, almonds, onion and tamari sauce. Add the water, mixing all ingredients well together to form a dough.
2. Refrigerate until chilled to make the dough easier to handle. Roll dough out thinly on a well floured board. Press sesame seeds into the dough and cut into strips 1^1/2 cm (^{3}/4 inch) wide, then cut each strip diagonally several times to make diamond shapes or cut with a biscuit cutter.
3. Place on a greased baking tray and bake at 180°C/350°F/gas mark 4 for 15–20 minutes, or until they are crisp and lightly browned.

MAKES 10

APPLE BREAD ROLLS

100 g (4 oz) silken tofu
150 ml (1/4 pint) So Good soya milk
2 eggs
50 g (2 oz) potato flour
50 g (2 oz) cornflour
50 g (2 oz) rice flour
50 g (2 oz) soya flour

1 tsp bicarbonate of soda
1/2 tsp cream of tartar
1/4 tsp tartaric acid
100 g (4 oz) grated apple
50 g (2 oz) soya margarine
1 tsp unrefined brown sugar
1 tbsp soya oil

1. Beat the tofu to a smooth purée with the So Good and eggs. This is best done in a liquidiser.
2. Mix all the dry ingredients for the rolls together with one tablespoon of soya oil.
3. Fold the flour mixture into the purée. Do not overmix and do not leave to stand at this point or you will lose the light structure of the bread dough.
4. Grease individual bun or muffin trays, and spoon the mixture into each.
5. Bake in a pre-heated oven at 220°C/425°F/gas mark 7 for 12–15 minutes.
6. Remove from the tray and cool on a wire rack.
7. Serve hot with sweet or savoury dishes.

Variation
Use 50 g (2 oz) grated carrot in place of the tofu.

MAKES 12

QUICK AND EASY FLAT BREAD

100 g (4 oz) tofu
150 ml (1/4 pint) So Good soya milk
1 egg
150 g (5 oz) rice flour
50 g (2 oz) cornflour

25 g (1 oz) soya flour
1 tsp bicarbonate of soda
1 tsp cream of tartar
1/2 tsp tartaric acid
1 tsp sugar
1 tbsp soya oil

1. Beat the tofu to a smooth purée with the So Good and egg. This is best done in a liquidiser.
2. Mix all the dry ingredients together with one tablespoon of oil.
3. Fold the flour mixture into the purée. Do not overmix and do not leave to stand at this point or you will lose the light structure of the bread dough.
4. Line a 25 cm (10 inch) square tray with baking parchment and spread the mixture evenly.

5. Bake in a preheated oven at 220°/425°/gas mark 7 for 30–40 minutes.
6. Serve warm or when a day or two old, toast lightly.

MAKES ONE 450 g (1 lb) LOAF

RICE, SOYA AND RAISIN BREAD

4 tbsp So Good soya milk
2 eggs
4 tbsp clear honey
4 tbsp soya oil
175 g (6 oz) rice flour

50 g (2 oz) soya flour
2 tsp baking powder
50 g (2 oz) organic raisins
25 g (1 oz) chopped nuts

1. Mix the So Good, eggs, honey and oil. Sieve the dry ingredients and gradually blend into the mixture. Stir in the raisins and nuts.
2. Pour into a greased loaf tin and leave to rest for 1 hour.
3. Bake in a pre-heated oven 180°C/350°F/gas mark 5 for 45 minutes.

MAKES ONE 450 g (1 lb) LOAF

wheat-free soya and linseed loaf

100 g (4 oz) soya flour
100 g (2 oz) potato flour
100 g (2 oz) rice flour
100 g (4 oz) Linusit Gold golden
  linseeds (whole)
100 g (4 oz) oat bran (or rice bran
  if on a gluten-free diet)
50 g (2 oz) sesame seeds
50 g (2 oz) sunflower seeds

225 g (8 oz) dried fruit of your
  choice e.g. raisins or organic
  apricots, chopped
2 pieces stem ginger (chopped very
  finely)
1/2 tsp each of nutmeg, cinnamon
  and ginger
900 ml (11/2 pints approximately)
  So Good soya milk

1. Mix all dry ingredients in a large bowl.
2. Pour the So Good over the dry ingredients and stir well.
3. Leave to stand for 1 hour.
4. Spoon the mixture into two 450 g (1 lb) or one 900 g (2 lb) greased loaf tins.
5. Bake at 175°C/350°F/gas mark 4 for approximately 1 to 1 1/2 hours or until firm on top.
6. Remove from tin(s) and leave to cool on a wire rack.
7. Serve warm or cold with butter, cheese, or fruit or nut spreads.

MAKES ONE 900 g (2 lb) LOAF

SEED BREAD

150 g (5 oz) soya flour
150 g (5 oz) rice flour
75 g (3 oz) potato flour
2 tsp cream of tartar
1 tsp bicarbonate of soda
75 g (3 oz) sunflower seeds

50 g (2 oz) sesame seeds
50 g (2 oz) golden linseeds
50 g (2 oz) caraway seeds
300 ml (1/2 pint) So Good soya milk
2 tsp clear honey

1. Sift flours, cream of tartar and bicarbonate of soda into a large bowl.
2. Add seeds to flour. Mix the honey and So Good and stir into the dry ingredients.
3. Pour mixture into a greased loaf tin and bake at 180°C/350°F/gas mark 4 for 40–45 minutes, or until the sides of the bread come away from the tin.

MAKES ONE 450 g (1 lb) LOAF

SUSSEX SOYA BREAD

Suitable for a bread maker.

3 eggs
2 tbsp unrefined brown sugar
3 tbsp walnut oil
2 tbsp Phyto Sprinkle (see page 183)
75 g (3 oz) soya flour
75 g (3 oz) cornflour
150 g (5 oz) rice flour

275 ml (10 fl oz) So Good soya milk
1 tbsp water
11/2 sachets fast-action dried yeast
1/2 tsp salt
2 heaped tsps wheat-free baking powder

1. Place all the ingredients in a food processor or mixing bowl and beat until smooth.
2. Pour mixture into the bread maker and programme it for 3 hours.
3. Remove the cooked bread from the bread maker and eat while warm or leave to cool.
4. Slice as conventional bread and serve with butter and pure fruit spread.

SOYA AND CORNBREAD

450 g (1 lb) cornmeal
100 g (4 oz) soya flour
1 tsp salt
1 tsp bicarbonate of soda
2 tsp baking powder

1 tbsp tahini or peanut butter
150 ml (1/4 pint) plain soya yogurt
300 ml (1/2 pint) So Good soya milk
juice of 1 lemon

1. Pre-heat the oven to 180°C/350°F/gas mark 4 and grease a 23 x 23-cm (9 x 9-inch) cake tin.
2. Mix the dry ingredients in a mixing bowl. In a separate bowl blend the remaining ingredients to an even consistency. Add this mixture to the dry mixture, stir well and pour into the greased tin.
3. Bake for 25–30 minutes. Cool in the tin then slice into quarters, lift out of the tin and serve warm.

SERVES 4

BUCKWHEAT SCONES

100 g (4 oz) silken tofu
1 egg
150 ml (1/4 pint) So Good soya milk
50 g (2 oz) buckwheat flour
50 g (2 oz) soya flour
100 g (4 oz) rice flour

25 g (1 oz) unrefined brown sugar
1 tsp bicarbonate of soda
1/2 tsp cream of tartar
50 g (2 oz) soya margarine
50 g (2 oz) organic sultanas
50 g (3 oz) chopped pecan nuts

1. Beat the tofu and egg with the So Good until well mixed.
2. Mix all the dry ingredients with the margarine until it resembles fine breadcrumbs.
3. Add the liquid ingredients to the flour and add the sultanas and nuts. Mix together until combined.
4. Spoon the mixture into greased bun or muffin tins and cook in a pre-heated oven at 220°C/425°F/gas mark 7 for 15–20 minutes.
5. Serve warm with butter and pure fruit spread.

MAKES 6

PASTRY

RICE AND POTATO PASTRY

75 g (3 oz) rice flour
50 g (2 oz) soya flour
75 g (3 oz) potato flour

50 g (2 oz) soya margarine
2 tbsp ground almonds
water

1. Put all the ingredients into a bowl and blend with a fork, adding sufficient water to mix. Knead well.
2. Roll out on greaseproof paper and use to line a flan dish.
3. Bake at 200°C/400°F/gas mark 6 until it is crisp and golden.

RYE SHORTCRUST PASTRY

225 g (8 oz) rye flour
pinch of salt

100 g (4 oz) soya margarine
2–3 tbsp cold water

1. Put the flour into a bowl and stir in the salt.
2. Rub in the margarine until the mixture resembles fine breadcrumbs. Add sufficient water to mix. Bake at 200°C/400°F/gas mark 6.

SHORTCRUST POTATO PASTRY

75 g (3 oz) rice flour
25 g (1 oz) soya flour
25 g (1 oz) cornflour

175 g (6 oz) cooked mashed potato
pinch of salt
100 g (4 oz) soya margarine

1. Beat the flours and salt into the potato, using a food processor if available. Add the margarine, and beat into the potato mixture.
2. Work the dough lightly into a ball, wrap in cling film and refrigerate for 30 minutes.
3. Knead the dough on a cold, floured (cornflour) surface until it is smooth and putty-like.
4. Refrigerate for another 30 minutes before rolling out on to the required shape. Roll between sheets of greaseproof paper as it is less likely to stick and break up. Use as required in any savoury recipe.

SHORTCRUST PASTRY

100 g (4 oz) silken tofu
1 egg yolk
2 tbsp water
75 g (3 oz) rice flour

75 g (3 oz) cornflour
1/2 tsp salt
60 g (21/2 oz) soya margarine
60g (21/2 oz) butter

1. Beat the tofu to a smooth purée with the egg yolk and water.
2. Put the flours and salt into a bowl, add the fat and mix well until it resembles fine breadcrumbs.
3. Mix in the tofu purée using a knife.
4. Work the dough lightly into a ball, wrap in clingfilm and refrigerate for 30 minutes.
5. Knead the dough on a cold, cornfloured surface until it is smooth and putty-like.
6. Refrigerate for another 30 minutes before rolling out into the desired shape. Use as required in any recipe.

NUTTY CRUST PASTRY

75 g (3 oz) rice flour
75 g (3 oz) ground almonds

75 g (3 oz) desiccated coconut
75 ml (3 fl oz) water

1. Combine all the ingredients and press into a greased flan dish. Bake for 15 minutes until lightly browned, or leave unbaked depending on the recipe.

BEVERAGES

BANANA SHAKE

1 l (2 pints) cold So Good soya milk
4 very ripe bananas
50 g (2 oz) ground almonds

1/4 tsp ground nutmeg
flaked almonds

1. Turn all the ingredients into a food blender or liquidiser and blend to a thick, frothy consistency.
2. Pour into chilled glasses and serve immediately with a garnish of flaked almonds.

SERVES 4

RHUBARB AND BLACKBERRY SMOOTHIE

450 g (1 lb) rhubarb, washed and trimmed
450 g (1 lb) blackberries, washed

1 l (2 pints) cold So Good soya milk
20 ice cubes, crushed
1/4 tsp vanilla essence

1. Place all the ingredients in a blender or food processor and mix until frothy.
2. Serve well chilled with extra ice cubes if wished.

SERVES 4

PEACH WHIZZ

4 ripe peaches
600 ml (1 pint) natural apple juice

1/2 tsp allspice
300 ml (1/2 pint) natural soya yogurt

1. Heat 600 ml (1 pint) of water in a saucepan and bring to a rapid boil. Use a slotted spoon to lower the peaches into the boiling water; leave them there for 30 seconds then lift them out and slip off the skins.
2. Slice the peaches in half and remove their stones. Turn the peach halves into a food processor with the apple juice and purée to an even consistency.
3. Pour this mixture into 4 large glasses and put them in the freezer for at least 1 hour until the juice is slushy.
4. Remove the glasses from the freezer and sprinkle a little of the all-spice over each serving.
5. Spoon one-quarter of the yogurt over each serving and stir the peach and yogurt vigorously. Serve at once.

SERVES 4

LEMON BARLEY WATER

100 g (4 oz) pearl barley   *peel of 1 organically grown lemon*
600 ml (1 pint) water   *15 ml (1 tbsp) unrefined sugar*

1. Measure the pearl barley into a saucepan and wash well in cold water. Drain and cover with the measured water. Place the pan over a medium heat and bring to a rapid boil. Boil for 55 minutes, until the barley softens and the liquid reduces.
2. Remove the pan from the heat. Place the lemon peel and sugar in a large, heat-proof bowl or jug. Strain the barley from the boiling liquid and pour the liquid over the lemon in the jug.
3. Stir well to dissolve the sugar then leave to cool. Pour into a sterilised bottle and use diluted as you would a squash.

MAKES APPROX. 600 ml (1 pint)

CRANBERRY CITRUS PUNCH

600 ml (1 pint) cranberry juice   *juice and rind of 1 lemon*
300 ml (1/2 pint) pure apple juice   *1 apple, chopped*
300 ml (1/2 pint) pure orange juice *1 orange, segmented and chopped*
300 ml (1/2 pint) water

1. Combine the juices with the water and add the chopped fruit. Chill in the fridge until icy cold, and top with crushed ice if wished.

SERVES 4

BANANA RAISIN WHIP

300 ml (1/2 pint) chilled So Good *100 g (4 oz) organic raisins*
  soya milk *1 tsp lemon juice*
2 chilled frozen bananas

Combine all the ingredients together in a blender and purée until smooth. Serve well chilled.

SERVES 2

FROTHY SOYA MILK WITH HONEY

600 ml (1 pint) chilled So Good *1 1/2 tbsp clear honey*
  soya milk

Combine the ingredients in a blender and purée for 1 minute at high speed until light and frothy. Serve immediately in chilled glasses, over ice if desired.

SERVES 2

CREAMY BANANA DATE SHAKE

75 ml (3 fl oz) pure apple juice *1 small banana (very ripe)*
50 g (2 oz) silken tofu *4 dates*

1. In a blender, combine the apple juice, tofu, banana and dates and blend until smooth.
2. Chill well before serving, adding ice cubes if desired.

SERVES 2

20
PHYTO PRODUCT ROUND-UP

PRODUCT DIRECTORY FOR THE UK

Milk and cream

Oat milk	
Sheep milk	
Evernat	Almond milk
	Hazelnut milk

Rice milk

Provamel	Rice Drink (organic)
Clearspring	Rice Dream natural/ vanilla (organic)

Soya milk

Bonsoy	Unsweetened (organic)
Granose (organic)	Unsweetened (organic)
Plamil	Unsweetened/sweetened (organic)
Prosoya	So Nice Unsweetened/ sweetened (organic)
Provamel ·	Sweetened (organic)
	Unsweetened (organic)
	Calcium enriched
	Honey and malt
	Vanilla
	Calcium and vitamin enriched
So Good	Original
	Low fat
Unisoy	Calcium and vitamin enriched
Valsoia	With almonds
Provamel	Soya Dream
Granose (organic)	Soya Creem

Flavoured milk

Prosoya	Vanilla/chocolate/ capuccino
Provamel	Strawberry/banana/ chocolate
So Good	Chocolate/vanilla
Vitasoy	Vanilla/chocolate/carob
Sunrise	Banana/chocolate/ strawberry

Cheese Substitutes

Toffuti	Cream cheese with garlic and herbs
SoyCo	Cheese slices
Biddy Merkins	Italian, flavoured
Bute Island Foods	Scheese
Kallo	Cream cheese with chives

Yogurts

Provamel	Yofu – strawberry/peach/ black cherry/vanilla (organic)
	Yofu – natural (organic)
Sojasun	Sojasun natural
Unisoy	Yogary – black cherry/ peach/raspberry
So Good	Yoghert – black cherry/ peach/pineapple/natural
Granovita	Yoghart – black cherry/ peach and apricot/ strawberry
Granose (organic)	Apricot/blackcurrant/ peach melba

Desserts

Granose	Non-dairy custard mix
Provamel	Vanilla Dessert
	Chocolate Dessert
	Hazelnut Dessert
Plamil	Soya rice pudding

Tofu ices

Swedish Glace	Pear/chocolate/strawberry/ vanilla
Toffuti	Chocolate/vanilla/ strawberry
Prosoya	

Meat alternatives

Dragonfly (organic)	Smoked tofu
	Unsmoked tofu
	Beany Burgers
	Beany Roasts
Cauldron	Smoked tofu
	Naturally smoked tofu
	Marinated tofu
	Vegetable burgers
	Chilli flavour tofu burgers
	Bean burgers
	Premium vegetarian sausages
	Lincolnshire vegetarian sausages
	Nut cutlets
Realeat	Veggie Mince/Veggie Steak
	Vege Banger (sausage mix)
	Vege Burger (burger mix)
	Fish cakes
	Veggie Bites
Clearspring	Silken tofu
Community Foods	Veggie Burgers
Suma	Bacon Bits
	Flavoured soya chunks/ mince
	Natural soya chunks/mince
Protoveg	Smokey Mince Snaps
	Minced soya and onion mix
	Unflavoured soya chunks
	Flavoured soya chunks
	Sosmix
	Burgamix
	Spicy Beanburger mix
Kitchen Garden (organic)	TVP (Textured Vegetable Protein) mince
	TVP curry
	TVP savoury

Just Wholefoods (organic)	TVP mince
Bio-culinair	Soya-sausage mix, burgers

Soya sauce and beans

Meridian	Tamari sauce (wheat-free)
	Shoyu sauce
Clearspring	Miso
	Shoyu
	Tamari
Sanchi	Miso
	Tamari
	Shoyu
Suma	Soya beans – dried
	Soya beans – tinned
Kitchen Garden (organic)	Soya beans – dried

Mayonnaise

Granovita	Soya mayonnaise – chilli/ garlic/lemon/plain
Kite	Amazannaise
Plamil	Soya 'mayonnaise'

Cereals

Holly Mills	Gluten-free muesli with soya flakes
Kallo (organic)	Puffed rice
Whole Earth (organic)	Cornflakes
Evernat (organic)	Cornflakes
Rapunzel (organic)	Spelt flakes
Mornflake	Toasted Oat Crunchy
Southern Harvest	Tropical muesli with soya and linseed

Bread and Pasta

Village Bakery	Chestnut and maize (gluten free)
Village Bakery (organic)	Rye bread
Allied Bakery	Burgen soya and linseed loaf
De-Rit (organic)	Rye honey loaf (with sultanas)
	Rye honey loaf (plain)
Sunny vale	Sourdough rye
Orgran	Rice and soya pasta (gluten-free)

Vogel — Soya and Linseed Loaf
Bio-Culinair — Brown and white bread mixes

Bread alternatives

Orgran — Corn crispbread
Corn crispbread with cracked pepper
Rice and corn crispbread
Rice and millet crispbread
Finn Crisp — Original Rye
Harvest Slims
Kallo (organic) — Rice cakes – plain/ sesame seeds/salted
Evernat (organic) — Rice cakes – plain/ sesame seeds/salted
De-Rit (organic) — Rice cakes – 4 grain cakes/plain/salted
Rye crispbread
Village Bakery (organic) — Oatcakes

Flours

Amaranth
Barley
Buckwheat
Carob flour
Corn
Cornmeal
Grain (chick pea)
Potato

Rye
Rice
Soya
Millet
Polenta
Sago
Quinoa

Healthfood bars

Tropical Wholefoods — Fruit bar
Banana flapjack
9 Bar — Organic Hemp bar
Pow Hemp and fruit bar
Wallaby Bar — Soya and rice fruit bar
Phytogenics — Prevacan bar
S P Shepherd Bar — Fruit and nut bars
Eat Natural — Fruit and nut bars
Sunita — Sesame bar
Holly Mills — Fruit bars
Equal Exchange — Sesame bar
D&D Chocolates (Dairy Free) — Chocolate bars
Novelties
Gluten free chocolates
Carob bars
Gift boxes
Plamil — Dairy free chocolate (organic)
Dairy free milk
Dairy free orange

PRODUCT LISTINGS FOR AUSTRALIA

Milk and soya

Goat milk
Suncoast 250 ml
NZ UHT
Oat milk
Sheep milk
Rice milk
Aussie Dream
Rice Delight
Rice Dream
Australia's Own
Soya Milk
Aussie Soya

So Good Lite
Australia's Own — natural
So Good — Now
Aussie strong Soya
So Natural
Aussie trim Soya
Soya Life
Berri soya
Soya King Natural
Bonsoy

Soylite
Goodlife
Sungold
Natures Soya
Vitalife
Soya Extra
Vitasoy
Soya Powders

Sanitarium	Soya Beans in tomato sauce
	TVP (textured vegetable protein)
	Tempah
	Thai Spicy Tofu
Pure Harvest	Silken Tofu
F.G. Roberts	Soya Compound
Healtheries	Soya wholegrain flakes
	Soya Grits
	Soya Flour
Sam Remo Macaroni	Soyaroni (Soya Pasta)

Yogurts

Attiki	Acidophilus, natural honey
Activ	Natural
Bulla	Reduced fat plan
Bornhoffen	Natural fruit flavours
Organic	All flavours
So Natural	Soya
Yoplus	Natural

Cheese substitutes

Lo Chol
Lite Chol
Soya Cheese
Tasty Lo Chol

Tofu ices

Tofu Gourmet (charioto)	
Amarina	All flavours

Meat Alternatives

Vege Hotdogs
Vege Party Franks
Vege Sausages
Notcorndogs
BBQ Soya Sausages

Soya Mince
Nutmeat
Vegelinks
Soya Beans in Tomato sauce
Vegetarian Rediburger
Vegetarian Sausages
Savoury lentils

Mayonnaise

Kraft	
Norganic	Golden Soya
Westbrae Soya	

Cereals

Uncle Toby's	Nut Feast
Abundant Earth	Gluten Free muesli
	Puffed corn/rice
Freedom foods	Gluten Free
Green's	Rice bran
Home Harvest	Millet puffs
	Brown rice puffs
Pure Harvest	Puffed corn
	Puffed millet
	Puffed rice

Bread

Gluten Free	Rite – Diet
Clarona	Multi Maize and Soya
Rice Bread	
Sourdough Soya	
Baker's Delight	Irish Soda Bread
	Linseed Soya
	Rye Swirl
Brumby's	Soya and Linseed
	Gluten Free
Buttercup	Soya and Linseed
Country Harvest	Gluten free
Gluten free High Fibre	
Country Life	Gluten free plain
	Gluten free sultana
	Hi – Soya
	Organic Rye
Defiance	Swiss Grain; Soya and Linseed
Tip Top	Barley Multigrain
Bornhoffen	Soya and Linseed
Vogel	Soya and Linseed
	Sunflower and Barley

Sandwich spreads

Melrose/ Freedom	Nut Spreads – Almond, Cashew, Pistachio, Hazelnut, Macadamia
Pure Harvest	Rice Syrup
Vital	Soya Lecithin

Bread alternatives

Burgen Bread	Soya-Lin Loaf
Orgran	Corn Crispbread
	Cruskits
Finn Crisp	Original Rye
Freedom Foods	Kalvi
Naturally Good	Soya carob
	Rice Crispbread
Ryvita	Dark rye
	Soya Lin

Rice Cakes

Sunfarm	Rice cakes
Trident	Corn
	Multigrain
	Sesame
Pure Harvest	Rice
Naturally Good	Soya Tri Grained
Freedom Foods	Soya Carob Orange
	Rice snax

Flours

Barley
Buckwheat
Carob flour
Cornmeal
Gluten flour
Potato flour
Rye flour
Rice flour
Soya
Linseed
Millet
Polenta
Sago

Terence Stamp	All-purpose wheat-free flour
Dove's Farm	Gluten-free flour mix

Biscuits

Arnott's	Sesame Wheat
Clarke's	Clusters- Apple and Walnut

	Cherry Ripple
	Nut and Fruit Ripple
Lane's	Captain's Table – sesame
Naytura's	Almond and Sesame
	Gluten Free

Health Food bars

Europe	Fruit and nut Bar
	Sesame Bar
Golden Days	Carob Cherry
	Sesame Snap
Go Natural; Be natural; Surene	Sesame Fruit and Nut
	Fruit and Nut Delight
	Nut Delight
Sun	Sesame
Alaska	Apple, Apricot Muesli Bar
Australia's Choice	Blackcurrant and Apple
Magic Apple Cookies	Sesame Slice Bar

Fruits canned and dried

Apple Rings

Glacé Fruit	Cherries
Ardmona	Canned apples
Farmland	Black Cherries
John West	Black Cherries in Syrup
SPC	Apples 100% Stewed
	Red Cherries in Syrup
Cottees	Fruit snacks

Tofu/Tempeh

Miso Liquid

Tofu	Nutrisoy
	Soya King
	Soyco
	Mori-Nu
Tempeh	Nutrisoy
	Nature's Miracle

Seeds

Linseeds
Sesame
Sunflowers
Aniseeds
Fennel
Pumpkin

PART THREE
APPENDICES

1

RECOMMENDED READING LIST

NOTE
UK, USA and A denote the following books are available in Great Britain, United States and Australia.

GENERAL HEALTH

Stewart M. & Stewart A. *Every Woman's Health Guide* Headline **UK A**

Stewart M. *Maryon Stewarts Zest for Life Plan* Headline **UK A**

Bradford, Nikki *The Well Women's Self-Help Book* Sidgwick and Jackson **UK**

Chaitow, Leon *Fibromyalgia and Muscle Pain* Thorsons **UK**

Dennerstein, Lorraine, Wood, Carl and Westmore, Ann *Hysterectomy – New Options and Advances* Oxford University Press, Melbourne **A**

Evans, Mark *A Guide to Herbal Remedies* The C W Daniel Co. Ltd **UK USA**

Graham, Judy *Evening Primrose Oil* Thorsons **UK**

Jacobs, Gill *Candida Albicans*, Optima **UK USA A**

Kilmartin, Angela *Understanding Cystitis* Arrow Books **UK A**

Liddell, L. *The Book of Massage* Ebury Press **UK**

Lockie, Dr Andrew and Geddes, Dr Nicola *The Women's Guide to Homeopathy, The Natural Way to a Healthier Life for Women*

Mayes, Kathleen *Osteoporosis* Thorsons **UK**

Melville, Arabella *Natural Hormone Health* Thorsons **UK USA A**

Nield, Larry *Escape from Tranquillisers and Sleeping Pills* Ebury Press **UK**

de Schepper, Luc, *Candida – Diet Against It*, Foulsham

Stevens, Chris *Alexander Technique* Vermilion **UK**

Stewart, Maryon *Healthy Parents, Healthy Baby* Headline **UK**

Stewart A. *Tired All The Time* Vermilion **UK A**

Trickett, Dr Shirley *Coming Off Tranquillisers* Thorsons **UK USA A** (Lothian Publishing Company)

Webb, Tony and Lang, Dr Tim *Food Irradiation: The Facts* Thorsons **UK**

Wescott, Patsy *Alternative Health for Women* Thorsons **UK**

DIET

Cox, Peter *The New Why You Didn't Need Meat* Bloomsbury **UK A**

Kenton, Susannah and Leslie *The New Raw Energy* Vermilion **UK A** (Doubleday Publishing Co.)

Vesanto M., Davis B., Harrison V., *Becoming Vegetarian* Macmillan Publishing, **USA UK**

Kirschmann, Gayla J. and Kirschman, John D. *Nutrition Almanac* (4th edn) Mc Graw-Hill Companies **UK USA**

Mabey, David and Gear, Alan and Jackie (eds) *Organic Consumer Guide/Food You Can Trust* Thorsons **UK**

STRESS

Dye, Jane *Aromatherapy for Women and Children* The C W Daniel Co. Ltd **UK USA**

Looker, Dr Terry and Gregson, Dr Olga *Stress Wise* Headway **UK**

Speight, Phyllis *Tranquillisation: The Non-Addictive Way* The C W Daniel Co. Ltd **UK USA**

RECIPE BOOKS

Berrydale, Michelle *Everyday Wheat and Gluten Free Cookery Book*

Cousins, Barbara *Cooking Without* HarperCollins Publisher **UK**

Doves Farm Gluten Free Baking

Holland, B., Unwin, I. D. and Buss, D. H. *Milk Products and Eggs* Royal Society of Chemistry, Ministry of Agriculture, Fisheries and Food (MAFF)

Hope, Simon *The Reluctant Vegetarian Cookbook* Heinemann: London **UK**

Leneman, Leah *The Single Vegan* Thorsons **UK**

Stamp, Terence and Buxton, Elizabeth *The Stamp Collection Cookbook* Ebury Press **UK**

Thomson, Peter *Gluten-Free Cookery: The Complete Guide For Gluten-Free or Wheat-Free Diets* Headway, Hodder & Stoughton **UK**

Vesanto M., Forest J., *Cooking Vegetarian* Macmillan Publishing **USA**

SMOKING

Carr, Allen *Easy Way to Stop Smoking* Penguin **UK**

DRUGS

Robson *Forbidden Drugs – Understanding Drugs and How People Take Them* Oxford University Press **UK**

Sanders and Myers *What Do You Know About Drugs?* Gloucester Press

EXERCISE

Cullum, Rodney and Mowbray, Lesley *YMCA Guide to Exercise to Music* (available from YMCA) **UK**

Myers, Clayton R. and Golding, Lawrence A. *The Ys Way to Physical Fitness* (available from YMCA) **UK**

2

USEFUL ADDRESSES

UK

Asset (Exercise Association)
4 Angel Gate,
City Road,
London EC1V 2PT
Tel: 020 7278 0811

Blackmores (UK)
The House of Blackmores,
37 Rothschild Road,
Chiswick,
London W4 5HT
Tel: 020 8987 8640

British Acupuncture Register and Directory
34 Alderney Street,
London SW1V 4UE
Tel: 020 7834 1012

British College of Naturopathy and Osteopathy
6 Netherhall Gardens,
London NW3 5RL
Tel: 020 7435 6464

British Diabetic Association
10 Queen Anne Street,
London W1M 0BD
Tel: 020 7323 1531

The British Homeopathic Association
27a Devonshire Street,
London W1N 1RJ
Tel: 020 7935 2163

British Osteopathic Association Clinic
8–10 Boston Place,
London NW1 6QH
Tel: 020 7262 1128

British School of Osteopathy Administration and Clinics
1–4 Suffolk Street,
London SW1Y 4HG
Tel: 020 7930 9254

British Wheel of Yoga
1 Hamilton Place,
Boston Road,
Sleaford,
Lincolnshire NG34 7ES
Tel: 01529 306851

Chiropractic Patients Association
8 Centre One,
Lysander Way,
Old Sarum Park,
Salisbury,
Wiltshire SP4 6BU
Tel: 01722 416027

The Council for Acupuncture
206–208 Latimer Road,
London W10 2RE
Tel: 020 8964 0222

The National Endometriosis Society
Suite 50,
Westminster Palace Gardens,
1–7 Artillery Road,
London SW1R 1RL
Tel: 020 7222 2781

The Faculty of Homeopathy
The Royal Homeopathic Hospital,
Hannemann House,
2 Powis Place,
Gt Ormond Street
London WC1N 3HT
Tel: 020 7837 9469

Food Watch International
Butts Pond Industrial Estate,
Sturminster Newton,
Dorset DT10 1AZ
Tel: 01258 73356

Friends of the Earth
26–28 Underwood Street,
London N1 7JQ
Tel: 020 7490 1555

Greenpeace
Canonbury Villas,
London N1 2PN
Tel: 020 7865 8200

**The Henry Doubleday Research
Association**
Ryton Gardens,
National Centre for Organic Gardening,
Ryton on Dunsmore,
Coventry CV8 3LG
Tel: 01203 303517

Homeopathic Development Foundation
19a Cavendish Square,
London W1M 9AD
Tel: 020 7629 3205

**International Federation of
Aromatherapists**
4 Eastmearn Road,
West Dulwich,
London SE21 8HA
Tel: 020 8742 2605

Lichter Pharma UK
Mere Park,
Dedmera Road,
Marlow,
Buckinghamshire SL7 1FJ
Tel: 01628 487780

Migraine Trust
45 Great Ormond Street,
London WC1 3HZ
Tel: 020 7278 2676

**The National Institute of Medical
Herbalists**
56 Longbrook Street,
Exeter EX4 6AN
Tel: 01392 426022

The National Osteoporosis Society
Barton Meade House,
PO Box 10,
Radstock,
Bath BA3 3YB
Tel: 01761 471771

Novogen UK
Suite 13,
Aron House,
6 Bardolph Road,
Richmond,
London TW9 2LS

Patients' Association
8 Guildford Street,
London WC1N 1DT
Tel: 020 7242 3460

**School of Phytotherapy
(Herbal Medicine)**
Bucksteep Manor,
Bodle Street Green,
Nr. Hailsham,
East Sussex BN27 4RJ
Tel: 01323 833812/4

The Shiatsu Society
31 Pullman Lane,
Godalming,
Surrey GU7 1XY
Tel: 01483 860 771

The Soil Association
Bristol House,
40–56 Victoria Street,
Bristol BS1 6BY
Tel: 0117 9290661

The Sports Council
16 Upper Woburn Place,
London WC1H 0QP
Tel: 020 7388 1277

Vegan Society
Donald Watson House,
7 Battle Road,
St Leonards-on-Sea,
East Sussex TN3Y 7AA
Tel: 01424 427393

Vegetarian Society
Parkdale,
Dunham Road,
Altrincham,
Cheshire WA14 4QG
Tel: 0161 928 0793

Women's Health
52 Featherstone Street,
London EC1Y 8RT
Tel: 020 7251 6580

**The Women's Nutritional Advisory
Service**
PO Box 268, Lewes,
East Sussex BN7 2QN
Tel: 01273 487366
http: //www.wnas.org.uk
email:wnas@wnas.org.uk

AUSTRALIA

ACT Cancer Society
15 Theodore Street,
Curtin 2605
Tel: 06 285 3070

Acupuncture Association of Australia
5 Albion Street,
Harris Park,
Sydney,
NSW 2150
Tel: 02 9633 9187

Adelaide Women's Community Health
64 Pennington Terrace,
North Adelaide
SA 5006
Tel: 08 267 5366

Anti-Cancer Council of Tasmania
13 Liverpool Street,
Hobart 7000
Tel: 03 6233 2030

**The Australian Consumers'
Association**
57 Carrington Rd,
Marrickville,
NSW 2044
Tel: 02 95773333
Fax: 02 95773377
email: ausconsumer@choice.com.au

Australian Nutrition Foundation
1–3 Derwent Street,
Glebe,
NSW 2037
Tel: 02 9552 3081

Australian Nutrition Foundation
PO Box 509,
Ashgrove,
Queensland 4060
Tel: 07 3366 7375

Blackmores Limited Advisory Service
23 Roseberry Street,
PO Box 258,
Balgowlah,
NSW 2093
Tel: 02 951 0111

Food Centre
140 Royal Street,
East Perth 6001
Tel: 09 235 6447

Liverpool Women's Health Centre
26 Bathurst Street,
Liverpool,
NSW 2170
Tel: 02 601 3555

National Heart Foundation
PO Box 2,
Woden 2606
Tel: 06 282 2144

**National Herbalists Association of
Australia**
PO Box 61,
Broadway,
NSW 2007
Tel: 02 9211 6437

Novogen Ltd
140 Wicks Road,
North Ryde,
NSW 2113
Tel: 61 2987 80055

NSW Cancer Council
153 Dowling Street,
Woolloomooloo,
NSW 2011
Tel: 02 9334 1933

Queensland Cancer Fund
553 Gregory Terrace,
Fortitude Valley 4006
Tel: 07 32258 2200

Women's Health Advisory Service
155 Eaglecreek Road,
Werombi 2570
NSW 2570
Tel: 046 531 445

NEW ZEALAND

The Association of Natural Therapies
PO Box 1055,
Palmerston North

Cancer Information Service
Auckland
Tel: 09 524 2628

Cancer Society
Christchurch
Tel: 03 379 5835

Health Alternative for Women
Room 101, Cranmer Centre,
PO Box 884,
Christchurch
Tel: 03 796 970

Heart Foundation
255 Madras Street,
Christchurch
Tel: 03 366 2112

Heart Foundation of New Zealand
17 Great South Road,
Greenlane,
Auckland
Tel: 09 524 6005

New Zealand Nutrition Foundation
PO Box 33/1409,
Takapuna,
Auckland
Tel: 09 9486 2036

Papakura Women's Centre
4 Opaneke Road,
Papakura,
Auckland
Tel: 08 267 5366

Tauranga Women's Centre
PO Box 368,
Tauranga
Tel: 783 530

West Auckland Women's Centre
PO Box 69116,
Glendene,
Auckland
Tel: 09 838 6381

Women's Health Collective
63 Ponsonby Road,
Ponsonby.
Auckland
Tel: 764 506

USEFUL ADDRESSES

Healthfood Companies and Manufacturers

UK

Cauldron Foods Ltd
Units 1–2,
Portishead Business Park,
Portishead,
Bristol
BS20 9BF
Tel: 01275 818448

Clear Springs Wholefoods Ltd
19A Acton Park Estate,
London
W3 7QE
Tel: 020 8749 1781

D & D Chocolates
261 Forest Road,
Loughborough
LE11 3HT
Tel: 01509 216400

Dragonfly Kitchen
Mardle Way,
Buckfastleigh,
Devon
TQ11 0NR
Tel: 01364 642700

Forever Green
3 Onslow House,
Castle Road,
Tunbridge Wells,
Kent
TN4 8BY
Tel: 01892 511652

GranoVita UK Ltd
Unit 2,
Everitt Close,
Denington Industrial Estate,
Wellingborough,
Northants
NN8 2QE
Tel: 01933 273717

Haldane Foods Ltd
Howards Way,
Newport Pagnell,
MK16 9PY
Tel: 01908 211311

Infinity Foods Ltd
67 Norway Street,
Portslade,
East Sussex
BN41 1AE
Tel: 01273 424060

Kallo Group Ltd
West Byfleet,
Surrey
KT14 6NF

Kite Wholefoods
Trecastle,
Brecon,
Wales
LD3 8UW

Meridian Foods Ltd
Corwen,
Clwyd
LL21 9RT
Tel: 01490 413151

Plamil Foods Ltd
Plamil House,
Bowles Well Gardens,
Folkestone,
Kent
CT19 6PQ
Tel: 01303 850588

Prosoya
2/3 Kingstone Park,
Nettlehill Road,
Houston Industrial Estate,
Livingstone
EH54 5DL
Tel: 01506 433777

Suma Wholefoods
Dean Clough,
Halifax
HX3 5AN
Tel: 01422 345513

Vandermoortele (UK) Ltd (Provamel)
Ashley House,
86–94 High Street,
Hounslow,
Middlesex
TW3 1NH
Tel: 020 8577 2727

The Village Bakery
Melmerby,
Penrith,
Cumbria
CA10 1HE
Tel: 01768 881515

Whole Earth Ltd
269 Portobello Road,
London
W11 1LR
Tel: 020 7243 0562

AUSTRALIA/NEW ZEALAND

Australia's Own Australian Natural Foods Holdings
PO Box 503, Carringbah,
NSW 2229
Tel: 02 526 2555
Fax: 02 525 5406

Bonsoy
Spiral Foods,
13 Cubitt St, Richmond,
Victoria 3121
Tel: 03 9429 8655
Fax: 03 9427 9207

Brumby's
PO Box 2106,
Clovelly West,
NSW 2031
Tel: 02 9326 3135
Fax: 02 9326 3137

Buttercup
23–25 Waterloo Road,
Ryde,
NSW 2112
Tel: 02 888 7177
Fax: 02 887 3222

Country Life Bakery
14 Kimberley Road,
Dandenong,
Victoria 3175
Tel: 03 9768 3077
Fax: 03 9768 3083

Healtheries
505 Mt Wellington Highway,
Mt Wellington,
New Zealand
Tel: 0 573 3730
Fax: 0 379 0489

Naturally Good Products
2/2 Clay Crescent,
Thomastown,
Victoria 3074
Tel: 03 9460 8050
Fax: 03 9460 4069

Pure Harvest
15 Ardena Crescent,
Brentleigh East,
Victoria 3165
Tel: 03 9579 3422
Fax: 03 9579 3312

Sanitarium Health Food Company
1 Sanitarium Drive,
Berkeley Vale
NSW 2261
Tel: 02 4348 7777
Fax: 02 4348 7786

So Natural
PO Box 203, Carringbah,
NSW 2229
Tel: 02 526 2555
Fax: 02 525 5406

Soya King
Tixama Ltd,
17 Elizabeth St, Campsie,
NSW 2194
Tel: 02 718 8255
Fax: 02 718 8772

Sungold
Australia Co-operative Foods Ltd,
Level 12/168 Walker Street,
North Sydney,
NSW 2060
Tel: 02 9905 5222
Fax: 02 9957 3530

Vitasoy
Melitta House of Coffee,
Unit 4, 801 Botany Road,
Botany,
NSW 2019
Tel: 02 316 9555
Fax: 02 316 9119

Vogels
Quality Bakers Australia,
18–52 Rosebank Avenue,
Clayton,
Victoria 3168
Tel: 03 9548 2511
Fax: 03 9547 7072

3

FURTHER HELP AND
TELEPHONE ADVICE LINES

If you would like to attend one of the WNAS clinics or need further details about our telephone and postal courses of treatment, you can write to the WNAS at the address below with an A5 self-addressed envelope and four separate first class stamps. Please state clearly what you require information about as we receive requests for so many different conditions.

The address to write to is:
Women's Nutritional Advisory Service, PO Box 268, Lewes, East Sussex, BN7 1QN

Or you can visit the WNAS website on www.wnas.org.uk   e-mail: wnas@wnas.org.uk

All clinic appointments are booked on 01273 487366

We also have a number of advice lines you may be interested in listening to:

Overcome PMS Naturally	09062 556600
The PMS Diet Line	09062 556601
Overcome Menopause Symptoms Naturally	09062 556602
The Menopause Diet Line	09062 556603
Beat Sugar Craving	09062 556604
Rediscover Your Zest for Life	09062 556605
Overcoming Breast Tenderness	09062 556606
Overcoming Period Pains Naturally	09062 556607
Get Fit for Pregnancy & Breastfeeding	09062 556608
Skin, Nails and Hair Signs of Deficiency	09062 556609
Improve Libido Naturally	09062 556610
Beat Irritable Bowel Syndrome	09062 556611
Overcome Fatigue	09062 556612
Beat Migraine Naturally	09062 556613
Overcome Ovulation Pain	09062 556614
The WNAS Advice Line Directory	09062 556615
Preventing Osteoporosis	09062 556614
Self-Help For Preventing Arthritis	09062 556645
Addressing Heart Disease Naturally	09062 556646
Overcoming Constipation Naturally	09062 556647
Detecting And Dealing With Allergies	09062 556648

The WNAS advice lines have been created to offer general advice to listeners on a range of health conditions. They are intended for information purposes only and are not specific for the individual. However, if you would like more detailed recommendations, you can enrol on a tailor-made nutritional programme, either over the telephone or at one of our clinics.

Calls are charged at 50p per minute and all proceeds are donated to the WNAS Charity Programme

4

MEDICAL REFERENCES

Standard References:

1. Davies, Dr Stephen & Stewart, Dr Alan, *Nutritional Medicine*, Pan Books, London 1987.
2. *Human Nutrition and Dietetics*, Passmore, R., & Eastwood, M.A., eighth edition, Churchill Livingstone, Edinburgh, 1986.
3. *Oxford Textbook of Medicine*, third edition, Weatherall, D.J., Ledingham, J.G.G. & Warrell, D.A. (eds) Oxford Medical Publications, Oxford, 1996.
4. *Nutritional Influences on Illness*, Werbach, Melvin R., Thorsons, 1989.
5. Messina Mark, Messina Virginia & Setchell Kenneth, *The Simple Soya Bean and Your Health*, Avery Publishing Group, New York, 1994.
6. Griffiths, K., Adlercreutz, H., Boyle, P., Denis, L., Nicholson, R.I., Morton, M.S. 'Nutrition and Cancer'. *ISIS Medical Media*. (1996).
7. Mindell, E., *Earl Mindell's Soy Miracle*, Fireside, New York, 1995.

Antiangiogenesis
(Inhibition of aberrant blood vessel development)

1. Adlercreutz, H., Goldin, B., Gorbach, S., Hockerstedt, K., Watanabe, S., Hamalainen, E., Markkanen, M., Makela, T., Wahala, K., Hasa, T. 'Soybean phytoestrogen intake and cancer risk'. *J Nutr*; 125(3 Suppl): 757S–770S. (1995).
2. Fotsis, T., Pepper, M., Adlercreutz, H., Fleischmann, G., Hase, T., Montesano, R., Schweigerer, L. 'Genistein, a dietary-derived inhibitor of *in vitro* angiogenesis'. *Proc Natl Acad Sci*; 90: 2690–2694. (1993).
3. Fotsis, T., Pepper, M., Adlercreutz, H., Hase, T., Montesano, R., Schweigerer, L. 'Genistein, a dietary ingested isoflavonoid, inhibits cell proliferation and *in vitro* angiogenesis'. *American Institute of Nutrition*; 1995(0022–3166/95): 790S–797S. (1995).
4. Peterson, G. 'Evaluation of the biochemical targets of genistein in tumor cells'. *J Nutr*; 125(3 Suppl): 784S–789S. (1995).

Anti-oxidant Effects

1. Cao, G.H., Sofic, E., Prior, R.L. 'Antioxidant and prooxidant behavior of flavonoids: Structure-activity relationships'. *Free Radic Biol Med*; 22(5): 749–760. (1997).
2. Degen, G.H. 'Interaction of phytoestrogens and other environmental estrogens with prostaglandin synthase *in vitro*'. *Journal of Steroid Biochemistry*; 35(3/4): 473–479. (1989).
3. Esaki, H., Onozaki, H., Kawakishi, S., Osawa, T. 'New antioxidant isolated from tempeh'. *J Agric Food Chem*; 44 (3): 696–700. (1996).
4. Wei, H., Qiuyin, C., Rahn, R.O. 'Inhibition of UV light- and Fento reaction-induced oxidative DNA damage by the soybean isoflavone genistein'. *Carcinogenesis*; 17(1): 73–77. (1996).

5. Jha, H.C., von Recklinghausen, G., Zilliken, F. 'Inhibition of *in vitro* microsomal lipid peroxidation by isoflavonoids'. *Biochemical Pharmacology*; 34(9): 1367–1369. (1985).
6. Ruiz-Larrea, M.B., Mohan, A.R., Paganga, G., Miller, N.J., Bolwell, G.P., Rice-Evans, C.A. 'Antioxidant activity of phytoestrogenic isoflavones'. *Free Radic Res*; 26(1): 63–70. (1997).
7. Wei, H., Wei, L., Frenkel, K., Bowen, R., Barnes, S. 'Inhibition of tumor promoter-induced hydrogen peroxide formation *in vitro* and *in vivo* by genistein'. *Nutr Cancer*; 20(1): 1–12. (1993).
8. Wei, H., Bowen, R., Cai, Q., Barnes, S., Wang, Y. 'Antioxidant and antipromotional effects of the soybean isoflavone genistein'. *Proc Soc Exp Bio Med*; 208 (Jan 1995): 124–130. (1995).

Breast Disease

1. Adlercreutz, H., Mousavi, Y., Hockerstedt, K. 'Diet and breast cancer'. *Acta Oncol*; 31(2): 175–181. (1992).
2. Adlercreutz, H., Mousavi, Y., Loukovaara, M., Hamalainen, E. 'Lignans, isoflavones, sex hormone metabolism and breast cancer'. In: Hochberg R.B., Naftolin F. (eds), *The New Biology of Steroid Hormones*. New York: Raven Press, 1991: 145–154.
3. Adlercreutz, H., Heikkinen, R., Woods, M., Fotsis, T., Dwyer, J.T., Goldin, B.R., Gorbach, S.L. 'Excretion of the lignans enterolactone and enterodiol and of equol in omnivorous and vegetarian postmenopausal women and in women with breast cancer'. *Lancet*; (Dec 11): 1295–1299. (1982).
4. Stevens, R.G. 'Dietary effects on breast cancer'. *Lancet*; 338 (July 20): (1991).
5. Adlercreutz, H. 'Diet, breast cancer, and sex hormone metabolism'. *Ann NY Acad Sci*; 595: 281–290. (1990).
6. Lee, H.P., Gourley, L., Duffy, S.W., Esteve, J., Lee, J., Day, N.E. 'Dietary effects on breast cancer risk in Singapore'. *Lancet*; 337: 1197–1200. (1991).
7. Mills, P.K., Beeson, W.L., Phillips, R.L., Fraser, G.E. 64:598–604). 'Prospective study of exogenous hormone use and breast cancer in Seventh-day Adventists'. *Cancer*; 64 (Aug 1): 591–597. (1989).
8. Martin, P.M., Horwitz, K.B., Ryan, D.S., McGuire, W.L. 'Phytoestrogen interaction with estrogen receptors in human breast cancer cells'. *Endocrinology*; 103(5): 1860–1867. (1978).
9. Verdeal, K., Brown, R.R., Richardson, T., Ryan, D.S. 'Affinity of phytoestrogens for estradiol-binding proteins and effect of coumestrol on growth of 17, 12-dimethyl-benz[a]anthracene-induced rat mammary tumors'. *JNCI*, 64(2): 285–290. (1980).
10. Baker, M. 'Evolution of regulation of steroid-mediated intercellular communication in vertebrates: insights from flavonoids, signals that mediate plant-rhizobia symbiosis'. *J Steroid Biochem Mol Biol*; 41(3–8): 301–308. (1992).

Cancer

1. Adlercreutz, H., Mousavi, Y., Clark, J., Hockerstedt, K., Hamalainen, E., Wahala, K., Makela, T., Hase, T. 'Dietary phytoestrogens and cancer: *in vitro* and *in vivo* studies'. *J Steroid Biochem Mol Biol*; 41(3–8): 331–337. (1992).
2. Adlercreutz, H., Goldin, B., Gorbach, S., Hockerstedt, K., Watanabe, S., Hamalainen, E., Markkanen, M., Makela, T., Wahala, K., Hase, T. 'Soybean phytoestrogen intake and cancer risk'. *J Nutr*; 124(3 Suppl): 757S–770S. (1995).

3. Adlercreutz, H. 'Phytoestrogens: epidemiology and a possible role in cancer protection'. *Environ Health Perspect*; 103(7): 103–112. (1995). (See Epidemiology)

4. Baghurst, P.G., Rohan, T.E. 'High fibre diets and reduced risk of breast cancer'. *J Cancer*; 1994: 173–176.

5. Barnes, S. 'Effect of genistein on *in vitro* and *in vivo* models of cancer'. *J Nutr, 125* (3 Suppl): 777S–783S. (1996).

6. Barnes, S., Peterson, G., Coward, L. 'Rationale for the use of genistein-containing soy matrices in chemoprevention trials for breast and prostate cancer'. *J Cell Biochem*: S22: 181–187. (1995).

7. Barnes, S., Peterson, G., Grubbs, C., Setchell, K. 'Potential role of dietary isoflavones in the prevention of cancer'. *Advances in Experimental Medicine & Biology*; 354: 135–147. (1994). In Jacobs, M.M. (ed) *Diet and Cancer: Markers, Prevention and Treatment*, New York, Plenum Press, 1994: 137–147.

8. Barnes, S., Sfakanios, J., Coward, L., Kirk, M. 'Soy isoflavonoids and cancer prevention – Underlying biochemical and pharmacological issues'. *Adv Exp Med Biol*; 401: 87–100. (1996).

9. Borina, F., Muti, P., Michell, A. *et al*. 'Serum sex hormone levels after menopause and subsequent breast cancer'. *J Nat Cancer Inst*. 1996; 88:291–296.

10. Bradley, D. 'A taste of soy keeps cancer at bay?' *New Scientist*, 1992:14.

11. Caile, E.E., Miraclememahill, H.L., Thus, M.J., Heath, C.W. 'Estrogen replacement therapy and risk of fatal colon cancer in prospective cohort of postmenopausal women'. *J Nat Cancer Inst* 1995; 87:517–523.

12. Cassidy, J.M., Zesmie, T.M., Chase, Y.H., Fern, M.A., Portvondo, N.E., Baird, W.M. 'Use of mammalian cell culture benzo (a) pyrene metabolism assay for the detection of potential anticarcinogens from natural products: inhibition of metabolism by biochanin A, an isoflavone from Trifolium pratense L.' *Cancer Res*; (1986) Nov 15; 48(22): 6257–6261.

13. Coward, L., Barnes, N.C., Setchell, K.D.R., Barnes, S. 'Genistein, daidzein and their B glycoside conjugates: Antitumor isoflavones in soybean foods from American and Asian diets'. *American Chemical Society*; 0021-8561/93/1441-1961: 1961–1967. (1993).

14. David, D.L., Bradlow, H.L., Wolff, M., Woodruff, T., Hoel, D.G., Anton-Culver, H. 'Medical hypothesis – xenoestrogens as preventable causes of breast cancer'. *Environ Health Perspect* 1993; 101: 373–374.

15. Franke, A., Custer, L., Cerna, C., Narala, K. 'Rapid HPLC analysis of dietary phytoestrogens from legumes and from hurine urine'. Molecular Carcinogenesis Program, Cancer Research Centre of Hawaii, Honolulu, Hawaii 96813, pp.18–23, 1995, vol. 208.

16. Franke, A.A. *et. al.* 'Phytoestrogens in human biomatrices including breast milk.' *Biochem Soc Trans.*, 1999; 27(2): 308–318.

17. Greenwald, P., Clifford, C., Pilch, S., Heimendinger, J., Kelloff, G. 'New directions in dietary studies in cancer: the National Cancer Institute'. *Adv Exp Med Biol*; 369: 229–239. (1995).

18. Griffiths, K, Adlercreutz, H., Boyle, P., Denis, L., Nicholson, R.I., Morton, M.S. 'Nutrition and Cancer'. *Oxford ISIS Medical Media* 1996.

19. Hawrylewicz, E., Zapata, J., Blair, W. 'Soya and experimental cancer: animal studies'. *J Nutr*; 125(3 Suppl): 698S–708S. (1995).

20. Hendrich, S., Lee, K., Xu, X., Wang, H., Murphy, P. 'Defining food components as new nutrients'. *J Nutr*; 124(9 Suppl): 1789S–1792S. (1995).

21. Jenab, M., Thompson, L.U. 'Influence of flaxseed and lignans on colon carcino-

genesis'. Proceedings of the 86th Annual Meeting of the American Association for Cancer Research Toronto, Ontario, Canada 1995: 114 (Abstr.).

22. Kennedy, A. 'The evidence for soybean products as cancer preventive agents'. *J Nutr*; 125(3 Suppl): 733S–743S. (1995).

23. Kondo, K., Tzuneizumi, K., Watanabe, T., Oishi, M. 'Induction of *in vitro* differentiation of mouse embryonal carcinoma (F9) cells by inhibitors of topoisomerases'. *Cancer Res*; 51: 5398–5404. (1991).

24. Kuo, S.M., 'Antiproliferative potency of structurally distinct dietary flavonoids on human colon cancer cells'. *Cancer Lett*; 110(1–2): 41–48. (1996).

25. Kuo, S.M., Summers, R. 'Dietary flavonoids induce apoptosis of colon cancer cells'. Proceedings of the American Association for Cancer Research, Toronto, Ontario, Canada 1992: 33:594 (Abstr.).

26. Le Marchand, L., Kolonel, L.N., Wilkens, L.R., Myers, B.C., Hirochata, T. 'Animal fat consumption and prostate cancer – A prospective study in Hawaii'. *Epidemiology*. 1994; 5: 276–282.

27. Lu, I.J., Anderson, K.E., Grady, J.J., Nagamani, M. 'Effects of soya consumption for one month on steroid hormones in premenopausal women: Implications for breast cancer risk reduction'. *Cancer Epidemiology, Biomarkers and Prevention*. 1996; 5(1): 63–70.

28. Makela, S., Poutanen, M., Lehtimaki, J., Kostian, M.L., Santti, R., Vihko, R. 'Estrogen-specific 17 beta-hydroxysteroid oxidoreductase type 1 (E.C. 1.1.1.62) as a possible target for the action of phytoestrogens'. *Proc Soc Exp Biol Med*; 208(1): 51–59. (1995).

29. Messina, M. 'Modern applications for an ancient bean: Soybeans and the prevention and treatment of chronic disease'. *J Nutr*; 125(3)(Suppl): 567S–569S. (1995).

30. Messina, M., Persky, V., Setchell, K., Barnes, S. 'Soy intake and cancer risk: a review of the *in vitro* and *in vivo* data'. *Nutr Cancer*; 21(2): 113–131. (1994).

31. Mills, P.K., Beeson, W.L., Phillips, R.L., Fraser, G.E. 'Cohort study of diet, lifestyle and prostate cancer in Adventist men'. *Cancer* 1989; 64:598–604.

32. Peterson, G., Barnes, S. 'Genistein inhibits both estrogen and growth factor stimulated proliferation of human breast cancer cells'. *Cell Growth Differ* 1996; 7:1347–1351.

33. Peterson, G., Barnes, S. 'Genistein inhibition of the growth of human breast cancer cells – Independence from estrogen receptors and the multi-drug resistance gene'. *Biochem Biophys Ros Commun* 1991; 179: 661–667.

34. Piontek, M.H., Hengels, K.J., Porschen, R., Strohmeyer, G. 'Antiproliferative effect of tyrosine kinase inhibitors in epidermal growth factor-stimulated growth of human gastric cancer cells'. *Anticancer Research*; 13(6A): 2119–2123. (1993).

35. Reinli, K., Block, G. 'Phytoestrogen content of foods – A compendium of literature values'. *Nutr Cancer*; 26(2): 123–148. (1996).

36. Rose, D. P. 'Diet, hormones, and cancer'. *Ann Rev Public Health*; 14: 1–17. (1993).

37. Serraino, M., Thompson, L.U. 'Flaxseed supplementation and early markers of colon carcinogenesis'. *Cancer*. 1993: 159–165.

38. Setchell, K.D.R., Borriello, S.P., Hulme, P., Kirk, D.N., Axelson, M. 'Nonsteroidal estrogens of dietary origin: possible roles in hormone-dependent disease'. *Am J Clini Nutr*: 40 (September): 569–578. (1984).

39. Severson, R.K., Nomura, A.M.Y., Grove, J.S., Stemmerman, G.N. 'A prospective study of demographics and prostate cancer among men of Japanese ancestry in Hawaii'. *Cancer Res* 1989; 49:1857–1860.

40. Steele, V., Pereira, M., Sigman, C., Kelloff, G. 'Cancer chemoprevention agent development strategies for genistein'. *J Nutr*; 125(3 Suppl): 713S–716S. (1995).

41. Thompson, L.U., Rickard, S.E., Orcheson, L.J., Seidi, M.M. 'Flaxseed and its lignan and oil components reduce mammary tumour growth at a late stage of carcinogenesis'. *Carcinogenesis* 1996; 17:1373–1376.

42. Thompson, L.U., Serraino, M. 'Lignans in flaxseed and breast and colon carcinogenesis'. *Proc Flax Inst US*. Fargo, ND, 1990: 30–35.

43. Vines, G. 'Cancer – Is Soya the Solution?' *New Scientist*, 1994:14–15.

44. Williams, M.C., Dickerson, J.W.D. 'Nutrition in Cancer – Some biochemical mechanisms'. *Nutrition Research Reviews*, 1990; 3:75–100.

45. Wiseman, H. 'Role of dietary phyto-oestrogens in the protection against cancer and heart disease'. *Biochem Soc Trans*; 24(3 PT 1): 795–800. (1996).

46. Xu, X.M., Thomas, M.L. 'Biphasic actions of estrogen on colon cancer cell growth possible ediation by high and low affinity estrogen binding sites'. *Endocrine* 1995: 3:661–665.

47. Yuan, J.M., Wang, Q.S., Rose, R.K., Henderson, B.E., Yu, M.C. 'Diet and breast cancer in Shanghai and Tianjin, China'. *Br J Cancer* 1995; 71:1353–1358.

Cholesterol

1. Anderson, J.W., Johnstone, B.M., Cook-Newell, M.E. 'Meta analysis of the effects of soy bean intake on serum lipids'. *New England Journal of Medicine*; 333(5):276–315. (1995).

2. Anthony, M.S., Clarkson, T.B., Hughes, C.L., Morgan, T.M., Burke, G.L. 'Soyabean isoflavones improve cardiovascular risk factors without affecting the reproductive system of peripubertal rhesus monkeys'. *American Institute of Nutrition*; 0022–3155/96:43–50. (1996).

3. Balmir, F., Staack, R., Jeffrey, E., Jimenez, M.D.B., Wang, L., Potter, S.M. 'An extract of soy flour influences serum cholesterol and thyroid hormones in rats and hamsters'. *J Nutr*; 126(12):3046–3053. (1996).

4. Cruz, M.L.A., Wong, W.W., Mimouni, F., Hachey, D.L., Setchell, K.D.R., Klein, P.D., Tsang, R.C. 'Effects of infant nutrition on cholesterol synthesis rates'. *Pediatric Research*; 35(2):135–140. (1994).

5. Goldberg, A.C. 'Perspectives on soy protein as a nonpharmacological approach for lowering cholesterol'. *J Nutr*; 125(3)(Suppl) 675S–678S. (1995).

6. Gooderham, M.H., Adlercreutz, H., Ojala, S.T., Waehaelae, K., Holub, B.J. 'A soy protein isolate rich in genistein and daidzein and its effects on plasma isoflavone concentrations, platelet aggregation, blood lipids and fatty acid composition of plasma phospholipid in normal men'. *J Nutr*; 126(8): 2000–2006, (1996).

7. Johnston, Ingeborg, M., James, R. 'Flaxseed (linseed) oil and the power of omega-3 – How to make nature's cholesterol fighters work for you'. *Good Health Guide*. 1990.

8. Kuppusamy, U.R., Das, N.P. 'Effects of flavonoids on cyclic AMP phosphodiesterase and lipid mobilization in rat adipocytes'. *Biochemical Pharmacology*; 44(7): 1307–1315. (1992).

9. Potter, S.M. 'Overview of proposed mechanisms for the hypocholesterolemic effect of soy'. *J Nutr*; 125(Suppl 3): 606S–611S. (1995).

10. Sharma, R.D. 'Effect of various isoflavones on lipid levels in triton-treated rats'. *Atherosclerosis*; 33: 371–375. (1979).

11. Sharma, R.D. 'Isoflavones and hypercholesterolemia in rats'. *Lipids*; 14(6): 535–540. (1979).

12. Siddiqui, M.T. 'Hypolipidemic principles of *Cicer Arietinum*: Biochanin-A and formononetin'. *Lipids*; 11(3): 243–246. (1975).

Diabetes

1. Anderson, J.W., Hanna, T.J., Fanti, P. 'Soy Protein and Protection from Diabetic Kidney Disease.' Third International Symposium on the Role of Soy in Preventing and Treating Chronic Disease, Washington D.C. 30 Oct to 3 Nov, 1999. Abstract.
2. Coelingh Bennink, H.J.T., Schreurs, W.H.P., 'Improvement of oral glucose tolerance in gestational diabetes by pyridoxine'. *British Medical Journal*, 1975;3;13–15.
3. Hanna, T.J., Fanti, P., Anderson, J.W. 'Beneficial Effects of Soy Protein on Renal Function in Type 1 Diabetic Patients at Risk for Nephropathy.' Third International Symposium on the Role of Soy in Preventing and Treating Chronic Disease, Washington D.C. 30 Oct to 3 Nov, 1999. Abstract.
4. McNair *et al.* 'Hypomagnesemia: A risk factor in diabetic retinopathy'. *Diabetes*, 1978;27:1075–1077.
5. Moles, K.W., McMullen, J.K., 'Insulin resistance and hypomagnesaemia, case report'. *British Medical Journal*, 1982;285:262.

Epidemiology

1. Adlercreutz, H. 'Phytoestrogens: Epidemiology and a possible role in cancer prevention'. *Environ Health Perspect*; 103(7): 103–112. (1995).
2. Key, T.J.A., Pike, M.C. 'The Role of Oestrogens and Progestogens in the epidemiology and prevention of breast cancer'. *Eur J Cancer Clin Oncol*; 24(1): 29–43. (1988).
3. Persky, V., Van Horn, L. 'Epidemiology of soy and cancer: Perspectives and directions'. *J Nutr*: 125: 709S–712S. (1995).

Fatigue

1. Behan, P., Goldberg, G., Mowbray, J.F. 'Post-viral fatigue syndrome'. *British Medical Bulletin*, 47 No 4. (1991).
2. Jenkins, R., and Mowbray, W. (eds) *Post-Viral Fatigue Syndrome*. John Wiley & Sons, Chichester, UK, 1990.
3. Manu, P., Lane, T.J., Matthews, D.A. 'The frequency of chronic fatigue syndrome in patients with persistent fatigue'. *Annals of International Medicine*, 1988; 109: 554.
4. Stewart, Dr A. *Tired All The Time*. Vermilion, London, 1996.

General

1. Adlercreutz, H., Fotsis, T., Bannwart, C. *et al.* 'Assay of lignans and phytoestrogens in urine of women and in cow milk by GC/ MS (SIM)'. In Todd, J.F.J. (ed), *Advances in Mass Spectometry-85: Proceedings of the 10th International Mass Spectometry Conference, Chichester*, John Wiley, 1986, 661–662.
2. Hutchins, A.M., Lampa, J.W., Martini, M.S., Campbell, D.R., Stavin, J.L. 'Vegetables, fruits and legumes – Effect on urinary isoflavonoid phytoestrogen and lignan excretion'. *J Am Diet Assoc*; 1995:95: 769–774.
3. Rosenblum, E.R., Van Thiel, D.H., Campbell, I.M., Eagon, P.K., Gavaier, J.S. 'Separation and identification of phytoestrogen compounds isolated from bourbon'. *Alcohol* 1987; Suppl 1:551–555.
4. 'The Realeat Survey 1984–1997: Changing Attitudes to Meat Consumption'. The Gallup Organisation.

5. 'Genetic Engineering: Too Good to go wrong?' Greenpeace UK, October (1997).
6. 'Neighbours from Hell II', Meridian Production. (1998).

Ischaemic heart disease

1. De Keyser, J., De Kippel, N., Merkx, H., Vervaek, M., Herroelen, L. 'Serum concentrations of vitamins A and E and early outcome after ischaemic stroke'. *Lancet.* 1992; 339:1562–1565.
2. Haq, I.U., Jackson, P.R., Yeo, W.W., Ramsay, L.E. 'Sheffield risk and treatment table for cholesterol lowering for primary prevention of coronary heart disease'. *Lancet* 1995; 346:1467–1471.
3. Platinan, P., Rimm, E., Korhonan, P., *et al.* 'Intake of dietary fiber and risk of coronary heart disease in a cohort of Finnish men: The ATBC study'. *Circulation* 1996 94: 2720–2727.
4, Stampfer, M.J., Rimm, E.B. 'Epidemiological evidence for vitamin E in the prevention of cardiovascular disease'. *American Journal of Nutrition.* 1995; 62(Suppl)1365S–1369S.

Genistein

1. Barnes, S., Peterson, T. 'Biochemical targets of the isoflavone genistein in tumor cell lines'. *Proc Soc Exp Biol Med;* 208(1): 103–108. (1995).
2. Barnes, S. 'Effect of genistein on *in vitro* and *in vivo* models of cancer'. *J Nutr;* 125(3 Suppl): 777S–783S. (1995).
3. Barnes, S., Peterson, G., Coward, L., 'Rationale for the use of genistein containing soy matrices in chemoprevention trials for breast and prostate cancer'. *J Cell Biochem;* S22: 181–187. (1995).
4. Buckley, A.R., Buckley, D., Gout, P.W., Liang, H., Rao, Y.P., Blake, M.J. 'Inhibition by genistein of prolactin-induced Nb2 lymphoma cell mitogenesis'. *Mol Cell Endocrinol;* 98(1): 17–25. (1993).
5. Carlo-Stella, C., Regazzi, E., Garau, D., Mangoni, L., Rizzo, M.T., Bonati, A., Dotti, G., Almici, C., Rizzoli, V. 'Effect of the protein tyrosine kinase inhibitor genistein on normal and leukaemic haemopoietic progenitor cells'. *Br J Haematol;* 93(3): 551–557. (1996).
6. Carlo-Stella, C., Dotti, G., Mangoni, L., Regazzi, E., Garau, D., Bonati, A., Almici, C., Sammarelli, G., Savoldo, B., Rizzo, M.T. 'Selection of myeloid pro- genitors lacking BCR/ABL mRNA in chronic myelogenous leukemia patients after *in vitro* treatment with the tyrosine kinase inhibitor genistein'. *Blood;* 88(8): 3091–3100. (1996).
7. Castro, A.F., Altenberg, G.A. 'Inhibition of drug transport by genistein in multidrug-resistant cells expressing P-glycoprotein'. *Biochem Pharmacol;* 53(1): 89–93. (1997).
8. Constantinou, A., Kiguchi, K., Huberman, E. 'Induction of differentiation and DNA strand breakage in human HL-60 and K-562 leukemia cells by genistein'. *Cancer Res;* 50: 2618–2624. (1990).
9. Diener, M., Hug, F. 'Modulation of C1-secretion in rat distal colon by genistein, a protein tyrosine kinase inhibitor'. *Eur J Pharmacol;* 299(1–3): 161–170. (1996).
10. Dwivedi, C., Zhang, Y., Jensen, H.J., Singh, K.K. 'Effects of genistein on skin tumor development in mice'. *Biochem Arch;* 12(4): 273–276. (1996).
11. Finlay, G., Holdaway, K., Baguley, B. 'Comparison of the effects of genistein and amsacrine on leukemia cell proliferation'. *Oncology Research;* 6(1): 33–37. (1994).
12. Fukutake, M., Takahashi, M., Ishida, K., Kawamura, H., Sugimura, T., Wakabayashi, K. 'Quantification of genistein and genistin in soybeans and soybean product'. *Food Chem Toxicol;* 34(5): 457–461. (1996).

13. Kanatani, Y., Kasukabe, T., Hozumi, M., Motoyoshi, K., Nagata, N., Honma, Y. 'Genistein exhibits preferential cytotoxicity to a leukemogenic variant but induces differentiation of a non-leukemogenic variant of the mouse monocytic leukemia Mm cell line'. *Leuk Res*; 17(10): 847–853. (1993).

14. Keppens, S. 'Effect of genistein on both basal and glucagon-induced levels of cAMP in rat hepatocytes'. *Biochem Pharmacol*; 50(8): 1303–1304. (1995).

15. Levy, J.R., Faber, K.A., Ayyash, L., Hughes, C.L. 'The effect of prenatal exposure to the phytoestrogen genistein on sexual differentiation in rats'. *Proceedings of the Society for Experimental Biology & Medicine*; 208:60–66. (1995).

16. Matsukawa, Y., Marui, N., Sakai, I., Satomi, Y., Yoshida, M., Matsumoto, K., Nishino, H., Aoike, A. 'Genistein arrests cell cycle progression at G2-M'. *Cancer Res*; 53: 1328–1331. (1993).

17. Mousavi, Y., Adlercreutz, H. 'Genistein is an effective stimulator of sex hormone-binding globulin production in hepatocarcinoma human liver cancer cells and suppresses proliferation of these cells in culture'. *Steroids*; 58(7): 301–304. (1993).

18. Nishio, K., Miura, K., Ohira, T., Heike, Y., Saijo, N. 'Genistein, a tyrosine kinase inhibitor, decreased the affinity of p56lck to beta-chain of interleukin-2 receptor in human natural killer (NK)-rich cells and decreased NK-mediated cytotoxicity'. *Proc Soc Exp Biol Med*; 207(2): 227–233. (1994).

19. Peterson, T.G., Coward, L., Kirk, M., Falany, C.N., Barnes, S. 'The role of metabolism in mammary cell growth inhibition by the isoflavones genistein and biochanin A.' Dept of Pharmacology, University of Alabama at Birmingham, 35294, USA. *Carcinogenesis* (1996), Sept, 17(9): 1861–1869.

20. Reenstra, V.W., Yurko-Mauro, K., Dam, A., Raman, S., Shorten, S. 'CFTR chloride channel activation by genistein: The role of serine/threonine protein phosphatases'. *Am J Physiol Cell Physiol*; 271(2): C650–C657. (1996).

21. Steele, V., Pereira, M., Sigman, C., Kelloff, G. 'Cancer chemoprevention agent development strategies for genistein'. *J Nutr*; 125(3 Suppl): 713S–716S. (1995).

22. Stevens, M.F., McCall, C.J., Lelieveld, P., Alexander, P., Richter, A., Davies, D.E. 'Structural studies on bioactive compounds: Synthesis of polyhydroxylated 2-phenylbenzothiazoles and a comparison of their cytotoxicities and pharmacological properties with genistein and quercetin'. *Journal of Medicinal Chemistry*; 37: 1689–1695. (1994).

23. Takeda, Y., Nishio, K., Nutani, H., Saijo, N. 'Reversal of multidrug resistance by tyrosine-kinase inhibitors in a non-P-glycoprotein-mediated multidrug-resistant cell line'. *Int J Cancer*: 57(2): 229–239. (1994).

24. Takuma, T., Tajima, Y., Ichida, T. 'Effect of genistein on amylase release and protein tyrosine phosphorylation in parotid acinar cells'. *FEBS Lett*; 380(1–2): 83–86. (1996).

25. Traganos, F., Ardelt, B., Halko, N., Bruno, S., Darzynkiewicz, Z. 'Effects of genistein on the growth and cell cycle progression of normal human lymphocytes and human leukemic MOLT-4 and HL-60 cells'. *Cancer Res*; 52(22): 6200–6208. (1992).

26. Uckun, F.M., Evans, W.E., Forsyth, C.J., Waddick, K.G., Ahlgren, L.T., Chelstrom, L.M., Burkhardt, A., Bolen, J., Myers, D.E. 'Biotherapy of B-cell precursor leukemia by targeting genistein to CD19-associated tyrosine kinases'. *SCIENCE* 267 (10 February): 886–891. (1995).

27. Vera, J.C., Reyes, A.M., Carcamo, J.G., Velasquez, F.V., Rivas, C.I., Zhang, R.H., Strobel, P., Iribarren, R., Scher, H.I., Slebe, J.C. 'Genistein is a natural inhibitor of hexose and dehydroascorbic acid transport through the glucose transporter, GLUT 1'. *J Biol Chem*; 271(15): 8719–8724. (1996).

28. Versantvoort, C., Broxterman, H., Lankelma, J., Feller, N., Pinedo, H. 'Competitive inhibition by genistein and ATP dependence of daunorubicin transport in intact MRP overexpressing human small cell lung cancer cells'. *Biochem Pharmacol*; 48(6): 1129–1136. (1994).

29. Versantvoort, C.H., Rhodes, T., Twentyman, P.R. 'Acceleration of MR-associated efflux of rhodamine 123 by genistein and related compounds'. *Br J Cancer*; 74(12): 1949–1954. (1996).

30. Wang, T.T., Sathyamoorthy, N., Phang, J.M. 'Molecular effects of genistein on estrogen receptor mediated pathways'. *Carcinogenesis*; 17(2): 271–275. (1996).

31. Wei, H., Wei, L., Frenkel, K., Bowen, R., Barnes, S. 'Inhibition of tumor promoter-induced hydrogen peroxide formation *in vitro* and *in vivo* by genistein'. *Nutr Cancer*; 20(1): 1–12. (1993).

32. Yamamoto, S., Shimizu, K., Oonishi, I., Hasebe, K., Takamura, H., Inoue, T., Muraoka, K., Tani, T., Hashimoto, T., Yagi, M. 'Genistein suppresses cellular injury following hepatic ischemia/reperfusion'. *Transplant Proc*; 28 (2 PT 3): 1111–1115. (1996).

33. Yang, E.B., Wang, D.F., Mack, P., Cheng, L.Y. 'Genistein, a tyrosine kinase inhibitor, reduces EGF-induced EGF receptor internalization and degradation in human hepatoma HepG2 cells'. *Biochem Biophys Res Commun*; 224(2): 309–317. (1996).

34. Matsukawa, Y., Marui, N., Sakai, T., Satomi, Y., Yoshida, M., Matsumoto, K., Nishino, H., Aoike. 'Genistein arrests cell cycle progression at G_2-M. *Cancer Research*; 53:1328–1331. (1993).

Isoflavone pharmacokinetics, absorption, metabolism and excretion

1. Adlercreutz, H., Fotsis, T., Bannwart, C., Wahala, K., Makela, T., Brunow, G., Hasel, T. 'Determination of urinary lignans and phytoestrogen metabolites, potential antiestrogens and anticarcinogens, in urine of women on various habitual diets'. *J.Steroid Biochem*; 25(5B): 791–797. (1986).

2. Adlercreutz, H., Honjo, H., Higashi, A., Fotsis, T., Hamalainen, E., Hasegawa, T., Okada, H. 'Urinary excretion of lignans and isoflavonoid phytoestrogens in Japanese men and women consuming a traditional Japanese diet'. *Am J Clin Nutr*; 54:1093–1100. (1991).

3. Adlercreutz, H., Fotsis, T., Lampe, J., Wahala, K., Makela, T., Brunow, G., Hase, T. 'Quantitative determination of lignans and isoflavonoids in plasma of omnivorous and vegetarian women by isotope dilution gas chromatography-mass spectrometry'. *Scand J Clin Lab Invest Suppl*; 215: 5–18. (1993).

4. Adlercreutz, H. 'Diet and sex hormone metabolism'. In Rowland, I.R. (ed), *Nutrition, Toxicity, and Cancer*, Boston, London: CRC Press, 1991: 137–195.

5. Adlercreutz, H., Hockerstedt, K., Bannwart, C., Bloigu, S., Hamalainen, E., Fotsis, T., Ollus, A. 'Effect of dietary components, including lignans and phytoestrogens, on enterohepatic circulation and liver metabolism of estrogens and on sex hormone binding globulin (SHBG)'. *J Steroid Biochem*; 27(4–6): 1135–1144. (1987).

6. Bannwart, C., Adlercreutz, H., Wahala, K., Brunow, G., Hase, T. 'Isoflavonic phytoestrogens in humans, identification and metabolism'. Helsinki: European Association for Cancer Research. (1987):1.

7. Bannwart, C., Adlercreutz, H., Wahala, K., Brunow, G., Hase, T. 'Identification of the isoflavonic phytoestrogens formononetin and dihydrodaidzein in human urine'. 169: 169. (1987).

8. Batterham, T.J., Shutt, D.A., Hart, N.K., Braden, A.W.H., Tweeddale, H.J.

'Metabolism of intraruminally administered [4-14C]formononetin and [4-14C] biochanin A in sheep'. *Aust Agric Res*; 22: 131–138. (1971).

9. Chang, Y.C., Nair, M.G. 'Metabolism of daidzein and genistein by intestinal bacteria'. *Journal of Natural Products*; 58(12):1892–1896. (1995).

10. Chang, Y.C., Nair, M.G. 'Metabolites of daidzein and genistein and their biological activities'. *Journal of Natural Products*; 58(12) 1901–1905. (1995).

11. Dickinson, J.M., Smith, G.R., Randel, R.D., Pemberton, I.J. '*In vitro* metabolism of formononetin and biochanin A in bovine rumen fluid'. *J Anim Sci*; 66: 1969–1973. (1988).

12. Franke, A., Custer, L., Cerna, C., Narala, K. 'Rapid HPLC analysis of dietary phytoestrogens from legumes and from human urine'. *Proc Soc Exp Biol Med*; 208(1): 18–26. (1995).

13. Franke, A., Custer, U. 'Daidzein and genistein concentrations in human milk after soy consumption'. *Clin Chem*; 42(6 PT 1): 955–964. (1996).

14. Hamalainen, E., Korpela, J.T., Adlercreutz, H. 'Effect of oxytetracycline administration on intestinal metabolism of oestrogens and on plasma sex hormones in healthy men'. *Gut*; 28 : 439–445. (1987).

15. Joannou, G., Kelly, G., Reeder, A., Waring, M., Nelson, C., 'A urinary profile study of dietary phytoestrogens. The identification and mode of metabolism of new isoflavonoids'. *Journal of Steroid Biochemistry & Molecular Biology*; 54(3–4): 167–184. (1995).

16. Kelly, G.E., Joannou, G.E., Reeder, A.Y., Nelson, C., Waring, M.A. 'The variable metabolic response to dietary isoflavones in humans'. *Proc Soc Exp Bio Med*; 208: 40–43. (1995).

17. Kelly, G.E., Nelson, C., Waring, M.A., Joannou, G.E., Reeder, A.Y. 'Metabolites of dietary (soya) isoflavones in human urine'. *Clin Chim Acta*; 223: 9–22. (1993).

18. King, R., Broadbent, J.L., Head, R.J. 'Absorption and excretion of the soy isoflavone genistein in rats'. *J Nutrition*; 126: 176–182. (1996).

19. Lloyd-Davies, H., Hill, J.L. 'The effect of diet on the metabolism in sheep of the tritiated isoflavones formononetin and biochanin A'. *Aust J Agric Res*; 40: 157–163. (1989).

20. Lu, L.J.W., Lin, S.N., Grady, J.J., Nagamani, M., Anderson, K.E. 'Altered kinetics and extent of urinary daidzein and genistein excretion in women during chronic soya exposure. *Nutr Cancer*; 26(3): 289–302. (1996).

21. Lundh, T. 'Metabolism of estrogenic isoflavones in domestic animal'. *Proc Soc Exp Biol Med*; 208(1): 33–39.(1995).

22. Nilsson, A., Hill, J.L., Davids, H.L. 'An *in vitro* study of formononetin and biochanin A metabolism in rumen fluid from sheep'. *Biochim Biophys Acta*; 148: 92–98. (1967).

23. Setchell, K.D.R., Adlercreutz, H. 'Mammalian lignans and phytoestrogens. Recent studies on their formation, metabolism and biological role in health and disease'. In Rowland, I.R. (ed), *Role of the Gut Flora in Toxicity and Cancer*, San Diego: Academic Press Limited. (1988):315–345.

24. Sharma, R.D. 'Effect of various isoflavones on lipid levels in triton-treated rats'. *Atherosclerosis* 1979, Jul:33(3):371–375.

25. Shutt, D.A., Weston, R.H., Hogan, J.P. 'Quantitative aspects of phytoestrogen metabolism in sheep fed on subterranean clover (Trifolium subterraneum cultivar clare) or red clover (Trifolium pratense)'. *Aust J. Agric Res*; 21: 713–722. (1970).

26. Slavin, J.L. 'Phytoestrogens in breast milk – Another advantage of breast-feeding? *Clin Chem*; 42(6 PT 1): 841–842. (1996).

27. Xu, X., Harris, K.S., Wang, H.J., Murphy, P.A., Hendrich, S. 'Bioavailability of soyabean isoflavones depends upon gut microflora in women'. *Journal of Nutrition*; 125(9): 2307–2315. (1995).

28. Xu, X., Wang, H.J., Murphy, P.A., Cook, L., Hendrich, S. 'Daidzein is a more bioavailable soymilk isoflavone than is genistein in adult women'. *J.Nutr*; 124(6): 825–832. (1994).

Menopause

1. Albertazzi, Paola *et al.* 'The effect of dietary soy supplementation on hot flushes'. *Obstetrics and Gynecology*, January, 1998; 91(1):6–11. (Address: Paola Albertazzi, MRCOG, Menopause and Osteoporosis Center, University of Ferrara, Ferrara, Italy) 28948.

2. Adlercreutz, H., Mousavi, Y., Clark., J, Hockerstedt, K., Hamalainen, E., Wahala, K., Makela, T., Hase, T. 'Dietary phytoestrogens and cancer: *in vitro* and *in vivo* studies'. *J Steroid Biochem Mol Biol*; 41(3–8): 331–337. (1992).

3. Adlercreutz, H. *et al.* 'Dietary phytoestrogens and the menopause in Japan'. *Lancet* (1992); 339; 1233.

4. Armstrong, B., Brown, J., Clarke, H., Crooke, D., Hahnel, R., Masarei, J., Ratajczak, T. 'Diet and reproductive hormones: A study of vegetarian and non-vegetarian postmenopausal women'. *JNCI*; 67(4): 761–767. (1981).

5. Baird, D. *et al.* 'Dietary intervention study to assess oestrogenicity of dietary soy among post-menopausal women'. *J Clin End Met* (1995); 80:1685–1689.

6. Boulet, M., Oddens, B.J., Lehert, P., Vemer, H.M., Visser, A. 'Climacteric and menopause in seven south-east Asian countries'. *Maturitas*; 19: 157–176. (1994).

7. Brown, J.E., Kahn, E.S.E. 'Maternal nutrition and the outcome of pregnancy – A renaissance in research'. *Clin Perinatol* 1997; vol. 24, issue 2: 433.

8. Cassidy, A. *et al.* 'Biological effects of a diet of soy protein rich in isoflavones on the menstrual cycle of pre-menopausal women'. *Am J Nutr* 1994; 60: 333–340.

9. Chung, T.K., Yip, S.K., Lam, P., Chang, A.M., Haines, C.J. 'A randomized, double-blind, placebo-controlled, crossover study on the effect of oral oestradiol on acute menopausal symptoms'. Department of Obstetrics and Gynaecology, Prince of Wales Hospital, Shatin, New Territories, Hong Kong. 1996; 25(2): 115–123.

10. Cline, J.M., Paschoid, J.C., Anthony, M.S., Obasanjo, I.O., Adams, M.R. 'Effects of hormonal therapies and dietary soy phytoestrogens on vaginal sytology in surgically postmenopausal macaques'. *Fertil Steril* 1996; 65:1031–1035.

11. The Committee on the Toxicity of Chemicals in Food, Consumer Products and Environment (COT) and the Food Advisory Committee (FAC) report on soya-based infant formulae.

12. Cowan, M.M., Gregory, L.W. 'Responses of pre- and postmenopausal females to aerobic conditioning'. *Medical Science, Sports and Exercise*, 1985; 17: 138–143.

13. Dalais *et al.* 'The effects of phytooestrogens in post-menopausal women'. Submitted to *Maturitas* 1997.

14. Davies, S., Stewart, A. *Nutritional Medicine*, Pan Books, London, 1987.

15. Eden, J. 'Phytoestrogens and the menopause.' *Baillière's Clinical Endocrinology and Metabolism*, 1998: 12(4): 581–87.

16. Eden, J.A., Knight, D.C., Howes, J., Kelly, G.E. 'The effect of isoflavones on menopausal symptoms'. *Abstract*. (1996).

17. Egger, J. 'Psychoneurological aspects of food allergy'. *European Journal of Clinical Nutrition*, 1991: 45 (Suppl. 1), 35–45.

48. France, K., Schofield, M.J., Lee, C. 'Patterns and correlates of hormone replacement therapy use among middle-aged Australian women.' *Women's Health* 1997 Summer: 3(2):121–38

19. Goldin, B.R., Adlercreutz, H., Dwye, J.T., Swenson, L., Gorbach, S.L. 'Effect of diet on excretion of estrogens in pre- and postmenopausal women'. *Cancer Research*; 41: 3771–3773. (1981).

20. Greist, J.H., *et al.* 'Running as treatment for depression'. *Comprehensive Psychiatry*, 1979; 20: 41-523.

21. Haas, S., Schiff, I. 'Symptoms of oestrogen deficiency'. In *The Menopause*, Studd, J.W.W., Whitehead, M.I. (eds), Blackwell Scientific Publications, Oxford, 1988, 15–23.

22. Hunt, K., Vessey, M., McPherson, K. 'Mortality in a cohort of long-term users of hormone replacement therapy: An updated analysis'. *British Journal of Obstetrics and Gynaecology*, 1990; 97: 1080–1086.

23. Jacobs, H.S., Loeffler, F.E. 'Postmenopausal hormone replacement therapy'. *British Medical Journal*, 1992; 305:1403–1408.

24. Knight, D.C., Eden, J.A. 'A short review of the clinical effects of phytoestrogens'. *Obstetrics and Gynecology*. 1996; 87: 897–904.

25. Knight, D.C., Eden, J.A. 'Phytoestrogens – a short review'. *Maturitas*; 22: 167–175. (1995).

26. Knight, D., Wall, P.L., Eden, J.A. 'A Review of phytoestrogens and effects in relation to menopausal symptoms'. *Australian Journal of Nutrition and Dietetics*; 53: 5–11. (1996).

27. Lock, M. 'Contested meanings of the menopause'. *Lancet* 1991; 337 1270–1272.

28. McLaren, H.C. 'Vitamin E and the menopause'. *British Medical Journal*, 1949; Dec 17: 1378–1381.

29. MacLennan, A.H., Wilson, D.H., Taylor, A.W. 'Hormone replacement therapies in women at risk of cardiovascular disease and osteoporosis in South Australia in 1997.' *Med J Aust* 1999 Jun 7; 170(11): 524–7.

30. Martin, K.A., Freeman, M.W. 'Postmenopausal hormone replacement therapy'. *The New England Journal of Medicine*, 1993; 328: 1115–1117.

31. Murkies, A.L., Lombard, C., Strauss, B., Wilcox, G., Burger, H.G., Morton, M.S. 'Dietary flour supplementation decreases post-menopausal hot flushes: Effect of soya and wheat'. *Maturitas*. 1995; 51(3); 189–195.

32. Nachtigall, L.B., Nachtigall, M.J., Nachtigall, L.E. 'Nonprescription Alternatives to Hormone Replacement Therapy.' *The Female Patient* June 1999; Vol 24; 45–50.

33. Notelovitz, M. 'The non-hormonal management of the menopause'. In *The Modern Management of the Menopause*, Berg, G., Hammer, M. (eds), Parthenon Publishing, 1994.

34. Punnonen, R., Lukola, A. 'Oestrogen-like effect of ginseng'. *British Medical Journal*, 1980; 281: 110.

35. Richard, S.E., Thompson, L.U. 'Phytoestrogens and lignans – Effects on reproduction and chronic disease'. *ACS SYMP SER* 1997; vol. 662: 273–293.

36. Sheehan, D.M. 'Isoflavone content of breast milk and soya formulas – Benefits and risks'. *Clin Chem*. 1997; vol. 43, issue 5: 850.

37. Slavin, J. 'More information on phytoestrogens in breast milk'. *Clin Chem* 1997; vol. 43, issue 3:548–3549.

38. Slavin, J., Jacobs, D., Marquart, L. 'Whole grain consumption and chronic disease – Protective mechanisms'. *Nutr Cancer*. 1997; vol. 27, issue 1: 14–21.

39. Stewart, M. *Beat The Menopause Without HRT*, Headline, London, 1997.

40. Stewart, M., Stewart, Dr A. *Every Woman's Health Guide*, Headline, London, 1997.

41. Taylor, M. 'Alternatives to conventional hormone replacement'. *Complementary Therapy*, 1997; vol. 23: 514–532.

42. Wahlqvist, Gisela, W., Burger, H, Medley, C. 'Oestrogenic effects of plant foods in postmenopausal women'. *BMJ*. 1990; vol. 301: 905.

43. Watanabe, S., Adlercreutz, H., 'Pharmacokinetics of the soy phytoestrogens in human'. *Abstr Pap Amer Chem Soc*. 1997; vol. 43, issue Apr: 135-AGFD.

44. Whitehead, M. 'Treatments for menopausal and post menopausal problems: present and future'. *Baillière's Clinical Obstetrics and Gynaaecology*. 1996; 10(3): 515–530.

45. Wilbush, J., 'Climacteric disorders – Historical perspectives'. In *The Menopause*, Studd, J.W.W., Whitehead, M.I. (eds), Blackwell Scientific Publications, Oxford, 1988, 1–14.

46. Wilcox, G. *et al.* 'Oestrogenic effects of plant foods in postmenopausal women'. *British Medical Journal*, 1990; 301; 905–906.

47. Wilson, R.C.D. *Understanding HRT and the Menopause*, Consumers' Association, London, 1992.

48. Winston, J., Craig, PhD, R.D. 'Phytochemicals: guardians of our health'. *Journal of the American Dietetic Association*, 1997:97 (Supp. 2), 199–203.

49. Woods, Margo N. *et al.* 'Hormone levels during dietary changes in premenopausal African-American Women'. *Journal of the National Cancer Institute*. October 2, 1996; 88(19)1369–1374.

Obesity

Standard references plus:

1. Garrow, J.S. *Treat Obesity Seriously, A Clinical Manual*, Churchill Livingstone, 1981.

2. Stewart, M., Stewart, Dr A. *The Vitality Diet*, Optima, London 1992.

Oestrogenic effects

1. Alexander, G., Watson, R.H., 'The assay of oestrogenic activity of *Trifolium subterraneum L.* by increase in uterine weight in the spayed guinea pig'. ? 457–479. (1951).

2. Baker, M. 'Evolution of regulation of steroid-mediated intercellular communication in vertebrates: insights from flavonoids, signals that mediate plant-rhizobia symbiosis'. *J Steroid Biochem Mol Biol*; 41(3–8): 301–308. (1992).

3. Collins, B.M., McLachlan, J.A., Arnold, S.F. 'The estrogenic and antiestrogenic activities of phytochemicals with the human oestrogen receptor expressed in yeast' *Steroids* 1997, Apr; 62(4):365–372.

4. Guillette, L.J.J., Arnold, S.F., McLachlan, J.A. 'Ecoestrogens and embryos – Is there a scientific basis for concern?' *Animal Reproduction Science*; 42:13–24. (1996).

5. Markiewicz, L., Garey, J., Adlercreutz, H., Gurpide, E. 'In vitro bioassays of nonsteroidal phytoestrogens'. *J Steroid Biochem Mol Biol*; 45(5):399–405. (1993).

6. Martin, P.M., Horwitz, K.B., Ryan, D.S., McGuire, W.L. 'Phytoestrogen interaction with estrogen receptors in human breast cancer cells'. *Endocrinology*; 103(5):1860–1867. (1978).

7. Mathieson, R.A, Kitts, W.D. 'Binding of phytoestrogen and oestradiol-17B by cytoplasmic receptors in the pituitary gland and hypothalamus of the ewe'. *J Endocrinol*; 85:317–325. (1980).

8. Molteni, A., Brizio-Molteni, L., Persky, V. 'In vitro hormonal effects of soybean isoflavones'. *J Nutr*, 125(3 Suppl): 751S–756S. (1995).

9. Santell, R.C., Chang, Y.C., Nair, M.G., Helferich, W.G. 'Dietary genistein exerts estrogenic effects upon the uterus, mammary gland and the hypothalamic/pituitary axis in rats'. *J Nutr* 127 (2): 263–269. (1997).

10. Sathyamoorthy, N., Wang, T.T., Phang, J.M. 'Stimulation of pS2 expression by diet-derived compounds'. *Cancer Res* 54 (4): 957–961. (1994).

11. Shutt, D.A., Cox, R.I. 'Steroid and phytoestrogen binding to sheep uterine receptors *in vitro*'. *J Endocrinol*; 52: 299–310. (1972).

12. Tang, B.Y., Adams, N.R. 'Effect of equol on oestrogen receptors and on synthesis of DNA and protein in the immature rat uterus'. *J Endocrinol*; 85: 291–297. (1980).

13. Verdeal, K., Brown, R.R., Richardson, T., Ryan, D.S. 'Affinity of phytoestrogens for estradiol-binding proteins and effect of coumestrol on growth of 7, 12-dimethyl-benz[a]anthracene-induced rat mammary tumors'. *JNCI*, 64(2): 285. (1980).

14. Walker, S.K., Obst, D., Smith, G.P., Hall, G.P., Flavel, P.F. 'Reproductive performance of sheep grazing oestrogen pastures on Kangaroo Island, South Australia'. *Agric Rec*; 6(10): 16–18. (1979).

15. Wang, T.T., Sathyamoorthy, N., Phang, J.M. 'Molecular effects of genistein on estrogen receptor mediated pathways'. *Carcinogenesis*; 17(2): 271–275. (1996).

16. Wang, W., Tanaka, Y., Han, Z., Higuchi, C. 'Proliferative response of mammary glandular tissue to formononetin'. *Nutrition & Cancer*; 23(2): 131–140. (1995).

Oestrogens vs phytoestrogens

1. St Clair, R.W. 'Estrogens and atherosclerosis: phytoestrogens and selective estrogen receptor modulators.' *Curr Opin Lipidol*, 1998; 9(5): 457–63.

Osteoporosis

1. Arjmandi, B.H., Alekel, L., Hollis, B.W., Amin, D., Stacewicz-Sapuntzakis, M., Guo, P., Kukreja, S.C. 'Dietary soybean protein prevents bone loss in an ovariectomized rat model of osteoporosis'. *Human and Clinical Nutrition*; 0022–3166/96: 161–166. (1995).

2. Berg, G., Hammer, M. *The Modern Management of the Menopause*, Parthenon Publishing, 1994.

3. Buck, A.C., Smellie, W.S., Jenkins, A., Meddings, R., James, A., Horrobin, D. 'The treatment of idiopathic recurrent urolithiasis with fish oil and evening primrose oil – a double blind study'. Department of Urology, Glasgow Royal Infirmary, Glasgow, In press.

4. Blumsohn, A., *et al.* 'The effect of calcium supplementation on the circadian rhythm of bone resorption'. *Journal of Clinical Endocrinology and Metabolism*, vol. 79:730–735.

5. Dixon, A.St.J. 'The non-hormonal treatment of osteoporosis.' *British Medical Journal*, 1983; 286:999–1000.

6. Ettinger, B., Grady, D. 'The waning effect of postmenopausal women'. *British Medical Journal*, 1990; 301:905.

7. Fujita,T., Fukase, M. 'Comparison of osteoporosis and calcium intake between Japan and the United States'. *Proc Soc Exp Biol Med*; 200(2): 149–152. (1992).

8. Kanis, J. A., *et al.* 'Evidence of efficacy of drugs affecting bone metabolism in preventing hip fracture'. *British Medical Journal*, 1992; 305: 1124–1128.

9. Kao, P., Peng, F. 'How to reduce the risk factors of osteoporosis in Asia'. *Chung Hua I Hsueh Tsa Chih Taipei*; 55(3): 209–213. (1995).

10. Lee Alekel, D., St Germain, A., Peterson, C.T., Hanson, K., Stewart, J.W., Toda, T. 'Isoflavone-Rich Soy Protein Isolate Exerts Significant Bone-Sparing in the

Lumbar Spine of Perimenopausal Women.' Third International Symposium on the Role of Soy in Preventing and Treating Chronic Disease, Washington D.C. 30 Oct to 3 Nov, 1999. Abstract.

11. Liberman, U.A., *et al.* 'Effect of oral alendronate on bone mineral density and the incidence of fractures in post menopausal osteoporosis'. *The New England Journal of Medicine*, 1995; 333: 1437–1443.

12. Lindsay, R. 'The menopause and osteoporosis'. *Obstetrics and Gynecology*; 87(2) (Suppl):1 6S–19S. (1996).

13. Martin, D., Notelovitz, M. 'Effects of aerobic training on bone mineral density of postmenopausal women'. *Journal of Bone and Mineral Research*, 1993; 8: 931–936.

14. Messina, M. 'Modern applications for an ancient bean: soybeans and the prevention and treatment of chronic disease'. *J Nutr*; 125(3) (Suppl): 567S–569S. (1995).

15. Notelovitz, M. 'The non-hormonal management of the menopause'. In *The Modern Management of the Menopause*, Berg, G., Hammer, M. (eds), Parthenon Publishing, 1994.

16. Novogen Ltd. 'Clinical evidence that Novogen product protects against bone and heart disease.' Press Release, 24/9/99.

17. Peel, N., Eastell, R. 'Osteoporosis'. *British Medical Journal*, 1995; 310; 989–992.

18. Scheiber, M.D., Liu, J.H., Subbiah, M.T.R., Rebar, R.W., Setchell, K. 'Dietary Soy Isoflavones Favourably Influence Lipids and Bone Turnover in Healthy Postmenopausal Women.' Third International Symposium on the Role of Soy in Preventing and Treating Chronic Disease, Washington D.C. 30 Oct to 3 Nov, 1999. Abstract.

19. Studd, John W., Whitehead, Malcolm. *The Menopause*, Blackwell Scientific Publications, 1988.

20. Taunenari, T., Yamada, S., Kawakaisu, M., Negishi, H., Tsutsumi, M. 'Menopause-related changes in bone mineral density in Japanese women – a longitudinal study on lumbar spine and proximal femur'. *Calcif Tissue Int* 1995; 56:5–10.

21. Van Papendorp, D.H., Coetzer, H., Kruger, M.C. 'Biochemical profile of osteoporotic patients on essential fatty acid supplementation'. *Nutrition Research*, vol. 15: No. 3, 325–334.

22. Wilcox, G., *et al.* 'Oestrogenic effects of plant foods in postmenopausal women'. *British Medical Journal*, 1990; 301:905.

23. WHO Study Group. 'Assessment of fracture risk and its application to screening for postmenopausal osteoporosis'. *World Health Organ Rep Sor* 1994; 843:11–13.

Phytoestrogens

1. Adlercreutz, H., Hamalainen, E., Gorbach, S., Goldin, B. 'Dietary phytoestrogens and the menopause in Japan'. *Lancet* 1992. 339:1233.

2. Anderson, J.W., Johnstone, B.M., Cook-Newell, M.E. 'Metanalysis of the effects of soy protein intake on serum lipids'. *N Engl J Med* 1995; 333:276–282.

3. Bhaden, A.W.H., Thain, R.I., Shutt, D.A. 'Comparison of plasma phytoestrogen levels in sheep and cattle after feeding on fresh clover'. *Australian Journal of Agriculture*, Ret., 1971, 22 663.70.

4. Brzezinski, A., Adlercreutz, H., Shaoul, R., Shmuell, A., Reosier, A., Schenkor, J.G. 'Phytoestrogen-rich diet – a possible alternative for hormone replacement therapy'. Meeting of the North American Menopause Society, Chicago, IL. 1996 (Abstr.).

5. Brzezinski, A., Adlercreutz, H., Shaoul, R., *et al.* 'Short-term effects of phytoestrogen-rich diet on postmenopausal women'. *Menopause,* J North Am Menopause Soc (in press).

6. Dwyer, I.T., Goldin, B.R., Saul, N., Gualtieri, L., Barakat, S., Adlercreutz, H. 'Tofu and soy drinks contain phytoestrogens'. *J Am Diet Assoc* 1994: 94:739–743.

7. Joannou, G.E., Kelly, G.E., Reeder, A.Y., Waring, M., Nelson, C. 'A urinary profile study of dietary phytoestrogens. The identification and mode of metabolism of new isoflavonoids'. *Journal of Steroid Biochemistry and Molecular Biology.* 1995; 54(3–4): 167–184.

8. Johanna, T., Dwyer, D., Goldin, Barry R., Nora, Saul, Gualtieri, L., Barakat, S., Adlercreutz, H. 'Tofu and Soy Drinks'.

9. Kelly, G., Husband, A., Waring, M. 'Standardized red clover extract', Natural Product Research Consultants, 1998.

10. Knight, D.C., Eden, J.A. 'Phytoestrogens – a short review;. *Maturitas.* 1995; 22(3): 165–175.

11. Lein, L.L., Lein, E.J. 'Hormone therapy and phytoestrogens'. *Journal of Clinical Pharmacy and Therapeutics.* 1996; 21(2): 101–111.

12. Martin, M.E., Haourigui, M., Pelissero, C., Benassayag, C., Nunez, E.A. 'Interactions between phytoestrogens and human sex steroid binding protein'. *Life Sciences.* 1996; 58(5): 429–436.

13. Miksicek, R.J. 'Commonly occurring plant flavonoids have estrogenic activity'. *Molecular Pharmacology.* 1993; 44(1): 37–43.

14. Obormeyer, W.R., Warner, C., Casey, R.E., Musser, S. 'Flaxseed lignans isolation, metabolism and biological effects'. *FASEB J* 1993: 7 Abstract 4965.

15. Peollinger, L., Whitelaw, M., McGuire, J. *et al.* 'Regulation of dioxin receptor function by genistein and phytoantiestrogens'. Third International Conference on Phytoestrogens, Abstracts. Little Rock AR: National Center for Toxicological Research, 1995.

16. Potter, J.D., Steinmet, K. 'Vegetables, fruit and phytoestrogens as preventive agents'. Cancer Prevention Research Program, Fred Hutchinson Cancer Research Center, Seattle, Washington, USA. 1996; 139: 61–90.

17. Price, K.R., Fenwick, G.R. 'Naturally occurring oestrogens in foods – a review'. *Food Addict Contam* 1985; 2: 73–106.

18. Reinli, K., Block, G. 'Phytoestrogen content of foods, a compendium of literature values'. *Nutr Cancer,* 26(2):123–148. (1996).

19. Rosenblum, E.R., Campbell, I.M., Vanthiel, D.H., Gavaler, J.S. 'Isolation and identification of phytoestrogens from beer'. *Alcohol Clin Exp Res* 1992; 16:843–845

20. Setchell, K.D.R. 'Naturally occurring non-steroidal estrogens of dietary origin'. In McLachlan, A. (ed), *Estrogens in the Environment – Influences on Development,* Elsevier, New York,1985: 69–83.

21. Wang, H.J., Murphy, P.A. 'Isoflavone content in commercial soybean foods'. *J Agr Food Chem* 1994; 42:1666–1673.

Phytoestrogen content of foods

1. Adlercreutz, H. & Mazur, W. (1997) 'Phyto-oestrogens and Western Diseases.' The Finnish Medical Society DUODECIM, *Annals of Medicine* 29: 95–120.

2. Mazur, W. 'Phytoestrogen content in foods.' *Baillière's Clinical Endocrinology and Metabolism* 1998 Dec; 12(4): 729–42.

3. Tham, D. *et. al.* (1998) 'Potential Health Benefits of Dietary Phytoestrogens:

A Review of the Clinical, Epidemiological, and Mechanistic Evidence.' *Journal of Clinical Endocrinology and Metabolism* 83(7): 2223–2235.

4. USDA-Iowa State University Database on the Isoflavone Content of Foods – 1999. Website address: www.nal.usda.gov/fnic/foodcomp/data/isoflav/isoflav.html

Platelets

1. Filpeanu, C.M., Brallolu, E., Huhurez, G., Siatineanu, S., Baltatu, O., Branisteanu, D.D. 'Multiple effects of tyrosine kinase inhibitors on vascular smooth muscle contraction'. *Eur J Pharmacol* 1995; 281:29–35.

2. Furman, M.I., Grigoryev, D., Bray, P.F., Dise, K.R., Goldschmidt-Clermont, P.J. 'Platelet tyrosine kinases and fibrinogen receptor activation'. *Circ Res* 1994; 75:172–80.

3. Goplan, R., Gracias, D., Madhaven, M. 'Serum lipid and lipoprotein fractions in benzal grain and biochanin A induced alterations in atherosclerosis'. *Indian Heart Journal*, 1991 May:43(3):185–189.

4. Ozaki, Y., Yatomi, Y., Jinnal, Y., Kume, S. 'Effects of genistein a tyrosine kinase inhibitor on platelet functions – genistein attenuates thrombin-induced Ca2 mobilization in human platelets by affecting polyphosphainositide turn over'. *Biochem Pharmacol* 1993: 46 395–403.

Prostatic disease

1. Adlercreutz, H. 'Phytoestrogens: Epidemiology and a possible role in cancer protection'. *Environ Health Perspect*; 103(7)103–112. (1995).

2. Adlercreutz, H., Honjo, H., Higashi, A., Fotsis, T., Hamalainen, E., Hasegawa, T., Okada, H. 'Urinary excretion of lignans and isoflavonoid phytoestrogens in Japanese men and women consuming a traditional Japanese diet'. *Am J Clin Nutr*; 54: 1093–1100. (1991).

3. Adlercreutz, H., Markkanen, H., Watanabe, S. 'Plasma concentrations of phytoestrogens in Japanese men'. *Lancet*; 342: 1209–1210. (1993).

4. Barnes, S., Peterson, G., Coward, L. 'Rationale for the use of genistein-containing soya matrices in chemoprevention trials for breast and prostate cancer'. *J Cell Biochem*; S22:181–187. (1995).

5. Bergan, R., Kyle, E., Nguyen, P., Trepel, J., Ingul, C., Neckers, L. 'Genistein-stimulated adherence of prostate cancer cells is associated with the binding of focal adhesion kinase to beta-I-integrin'. *Clin Exp Metastasis*; 14(4): 389–398. (1996).

6. Buck, A.C. 'Phytotherapy for the prostate'. *Br J Urol*; 78(3): 325–336. (1996).

7. Evans, B., Griffiths, K., Morton, M. 'Inhibition of 5 alpha-reductase in genital skin fibroblasts and prostate tissue by dietary lignans and isoflavonoids'. *Journal of Endocrinology*; 147(2): 295–302. (1995).

8. Makela, S., Pylkkanen, L., Santti, R., Adlercreutz, H. 'Role of plant estrogens in normal and estrogen-related altered growth of the mouse prostate'. *EURO FOOD TOX III, Proc Effects of Food on the Immune and Hormonal Systems*; May: 135–139. (1991).

9. Makela, S., Santti, R., Salo, L., McLachlan, J.A. 'Phytoestrogens are partial estrogen agonists in the adult male mouse'. *Environ Health Perspect*; 103(Suppl 7): 123–127. (1995).

10. Mills, P.K., Beeson, W.L., Phillips, R.L., Fraser, G.E. 'Cohort study of diet, lifestyle and prostate cancer in Adventist men'. *Cancer*; 64: 598–604. (1989).

11. Naik, H.R. 'An *in vitro* and *in vivo* study of antitumor effects of genistein on hormone refractory prostate cancer'. *Anticancer Research*; 14(6B): 2617–2619. (1994).

12. Peterson, G., Barnes, S. 'Genistein and biochanin A inhibit the growth of human prostate cancer cells but not epidermal growth factor receptor tyrosine utophosphorylation'. *Prostate*; 22(4): 335–345. (1993).
13. Sharma, O.P., Adlercreutz, H., Strandberg, J.D., Zirkin, B.R., Coffery, D.S., Ewing, L.L. 'Soya of dietary source plays a preventive role against the pathogenesis of prostatisis in rats'. *J Steroid Biochem Mol Biol*; 43: 557–564. (1992).

Puberty

1. de Ridder, C.M., Thijssen, J.H.H., Van't Veer, P. *et al.* 'Dietary habits, sexual maturation and plasma hormones in pubertal girls – a longitudinal study'. *Am J Clin Nutr* 1991; 54: 805–813.

Stress

1. Guthrie, E., Creed, F., Dawson, D., Tomensen, B. 'A controlled trial of psychological treatment for the irritable bowel syndrome'. *Gastroenterology*. 1991; 100:450–457.
2. Harvey, R.F., Hinton, R.A., Gunary, R.M., Barry, R.E. 'Individual and group hypnotherapy in the treatment of refractory irritable bowel syndrome'. *Lancet*. 1989; 1:424–425.
3. Swedlund, J., Sjoden, L., Ottosson, J.O., Doteval, G. 'Controlled study of psychological treatment for the irritable bowel syndrome'. *Lancet*. 1983; 2:589–591.
4. Whorwell, P.J., Prior, A., Colgan, S.M. 'Hypnotherapy in severe irritable bowel syndrome: Further experience'. *Gut*. 1987; 28:423–425.

Toxicology

1. Anthony, M.S., Clarkson, T.B., Hughes, C.L., Morgan, T.M., Burke, G.L. 'Soybean isoflavones improve cardiovascular risk factors without affecting the reproductive system of peripubertal rhesus monkeys'. *American Institute of Nutrition*; 0022–3155/96:43–50. (1996).
2. Bartholomew, R.M., Ryan, D.S. 'Lack of mutagenicity of some phytoestrogens in the salmonella/mammalian microsome assay'. *Mutation Research*; 78(4): 317–321. (1980).
3. Chae, Y.H., Coffing, S.L., Cook, V.M., Ho, D.K., Cassidy, I.M., Baird, W.M. 'Effects of biochanin A on metabolism, DNA binding and mutagenicity of benzo(a)pyrene in mammaliam cell cultures'. *Carcinogenesis*; 12(11): 2001–2006. (1991).
4. Czeczot, H., Kustztelak, J.A. 'Study of the genotoxic potential of flavonoids using short term bacterial assays'. *Acta Biochimica Polonica*; 40 : 549–554. (1993).
5. Degen, G.H. 'Interaction of phytoestrogens and other environmental estrogens with prostaglandin synthesis *in vitro*'. *Journal of Steroid Biochemistry*; 35(3/4): 473–479. (1989).
6. Farmakalidis, E., Hathcock, J.N., Murphy, P.A. 'Oestrogenic potency of genistein and daidzin in mice'. *Fd Chem Toxic*; 23(8): 741–745. (1985).
7. Hughes, C.L. 'Phytochemical mimicry of reproductive hormones and modulation of herbivore fertility by phytoestrogens'. *Environ Health Perspect*; 78: 171–175. (1991).
8. Hughes. C.J., Kaldas, R., Weisinger, A., McCants, C., Basham, K. 'Acute and sub-acute effects of naturally occurring estrogens on luteinizing hormone secretion in the ovariectomized rat: Part 1'. *Reproductive Toxicology*; 5(2): 127–132. (1991).

9. Iguchi, T. 'Cellular effects of early exposure to sex hormones and antihormones'. *Int Rev Cytol*; 139: 1–57. (1992).

10. Levy, J.R., Faber, K.A., Ayyash, L., Hughes, C.L. 'The effect of parental exposure to the phytoestrogen genistein on sexual differentiation in rats'. *Proceeding of the Society for Experimental Biology and Medicine*; 208: 60–66. (1995).

11. Liener, I. 'Implications of antinutritional components in soybean foods'. Crit rev *Food Sci Nutr*; 34(1): 31–67. (1994).

12. Liener, I.E. 'Possible adverse effects of soybean anticarcinogens'. *Amercan Institute of Nutrition*; 0022–3166: 744S–750S. (1995).

13. Medlock, K.L., Branham, W.S., Sheehan, D.M. 'Effects of coumestrol and equol on the developing reproductive tract of the rat'. *Proc Soc Exp Bio Med*; 208: 67–71. (1995).

14. Murrill, W.B., Brown, N.M., Zhang, J.X., Manzolillo, P.A., Barnes, S., Lamartiniere, C.A. 'Prepubertal genistein exposure suppresses mammary cancer and enhances gland differentiation in rats'. *Carcinogenesis*; 17(7): 1451–1457. (1996).

15. Sharpe, R., Skakkebaek, N. 'Are oestrogens involved in the falling sperm counts and disorders of the male reproductive tract?' *Lancet*; 341(8857): 1392–1395. (1993).

16. Sheehan, D.M. 'The case for expanded phytoestrogen research'. *Proc Soc Exp Biol Med*; 208(1): 3–5. (1995).

17. Smith, C., Halliwell, B., Aruoma. 'Protection by albumin against the pro-oxidant actions of phenolic dietary components'. *Food and Chemical Toxicology*; 483–489. (1992).

18. Wang, W., Tanaka, Y., Han, Z., Higuchi, C. 'Proliferative response of mammary glandular tissue to formononetin'. *Nutrition and Cancer*; 23(2): 131–140. (1995).

19. Whitten, P.L., Naftolin, F. 'Dietary estrogens: A biologically active background for estrogen action'. In Hochberg, R., Naftolin, F. (eds), *The New Biology of Steroid Hormones*, Raven Press, New York, 1991: 155–167.

Vascular compliance (Reactivity)

1. Honore, E.K., Williams, J.K., Anthony, M.S., Clarkson, T.B. 'Soya isoflavones enhance coronary vascular reactivity in atherosclerotic female macaques'. *Fertu Steril*; 67(1): 148–54. (1997).

2. Low, A.M. 'Role of tyrosine kinase on Ca2+ entry and refilling of agonist-sensitive Ca2+ stores in vascular smooth muscles'. *Can J Physiol Pharmacol*; 74(3): 298–304. (1996).

3. Marczin, N., Papapetropoulos, A., Catravas, J. 'Tyrosine kinase inhibitors suppress endotoxin- and IL-1 beta-induced NO synthesis in aortic smooth muscle cells'. *Am J Physiol*; 265(3 PT 2): H1014–1018. (1993).

4. Smirnov, S., Aaronson, P. 'Inhibition of vascular smooth muscle cell K+ currents by tyrosine kinase inhibitors genistein and ST 638'. *Circ Res*; 76(2): 310–316. (1995).

5. Taskinen, P., Toth, M., Ruskoaho, H. 'Effects of genistein on cardiac contractile force and atrial natriuretic peptide secretion in the isolated perfused rat heart'. *Eur J Pharmacol*; 256(3): 251–261. (1994).

6. Yang, I.C.H., Cheng, T.H., Wang, F., Price, E.M., Hwang, T.C. 'Modulation of CFTR chloride channels by calyculin A and genistein'. *Am J Physiol Cell Physiol*; 272(1): C142–C155. (1997).

5

NUTRITIONAL CONTENT OF FOODS

Unless stated otherwise, foods listed are raw

Vitamin A – retinol
Micrograms per 100 g (3.5 oz)

Skimmed milk	1
Semi-skimmed milk	21
Grilled herring	49
Whole milk	52
Porridge made with milk	56
Cheddar cheese	325
Margarine	800
Butter	815
Lamb's liver	15,000

Vitamin B1 – thiamin
Milligrams per 100 g (3.5 oz)

Peaches	0.02
Cottage cheese	0.02
Cox's apple	0.03
Full-fat milk	0.04
Skimmed milk	0.04
Semi-skimmed milk	0.04
Cheddar cheese	0.04
Bananas	0.04
White grapes	0.04
French beans	0.04
Low-fat yogurt	0.05
Canteloupe melon	0.05
Tomato	0.06
Green peppers, raw	0.07
Boiled egg	0.08
Roast chicken	0.08
Grilled cod	0.08
Haddock, steamed	0.08
Roast turkey	0.09
Mackerel, cooked	0.09
Savoy cabbage, boiled	0.10
Oranges	0.10
Brussels sprouts	0.10
Lentils, boiled	0.11
Potatoes, new, boiled	0.11
Soya beans, boiled	0.12
Red peppers, raw	0.12
Steamed salmon	0.20
Corn	0.20
White spaghetti, boiled	0.21
Almonds	0.24
White self-raising flour	0.30
Plaice, steamed	0.30
Bacon, cooked	0.35
Walnuts	0.40
Wholemeal flour	0.47
Lamb's kidney	0.49
Brazil nuts	1.00
Cornflakes	1.00
Rice Krispies	1.00
Wheatgerm	2.01

Vitamin B2 – riboflavin
Milligrams per 100 g (3.5 oz)

Cabbage, boiled	0.01
Potatoes, boiled	0.01
Brown rice, boiled	0.02
Pear	0.03
Wholemeal spaghetti, boiled	0.03
White self-raising flour	0.03
Orange	0.04
Spinach, boiled in salted water	0.05
Baked beans	0.06
Banana	0.06
White bread	0.06
Green peppers, raw	0.08
Lentils, boiled	0.08
Hovis	0.09

Soya beans, boiled	0.09
Wholemeal bread	0.09
Wholemeal flour	0.09
Peanuts	0.10
Baked salmon	0.11
Red peppers, raw	0.15
Full-fat milk	0.17
Avocado	0.18
Grilled herring	0.18
Semi-skimmed milk	0.18
Roast chicken	0.19
Roast turkey	0.21
Cottage cheese	0.26
Soya flour	0.31
Boiled prawns	0.34
Boiled egg	0.35
Topside of beef, cooked	0.35
Leg of lamb, cooked	0.38
Cheddar cheese	0.40
Muesli	0.70
Almonds	0.75
Cornflakes	1.50
Rice Krispies	1.50

Vitamin B3 – niacin
Milligrams per 100 g (3.5 oz)

Boiled egg	0.07
Cheddar cheese	0.07
Full-fat milk	0.08
Skimmed milk	0.09
Semi-skimmed milk	0.09
Cottage cheese	0.13
Cox's apple	0.20
Cabbage, boiled	0.30
Orange	0.40
Baked beans	0.50
Potatoes, boiled	0.50
Soya beans, boiled	0.50
Lentils, boiled	0.60
Banana	0.70
Tomato	1.00
Avocado	1.10
Green peppers, raw	1.10
Brown rice	1.30
Wholemeal spaghetti, boiled	1.30
White self-raising flour	1.50

Grilled cod	1.70
White bread	1.70
Soya flour	2.00
Red peppers, raw	2.20
Almonds	3.10
Grilled herring	4.00
Wholemeal bread	4.10
Hovis	4.20
Wholemeal flour	5.70
Muesli	6.50
Topside of beef, cooked	6.50
Leg of lamb, cooked	6.60
Baked salmon	7.00
Roast chicken	8.20
Roast turkey	8.50
Boiled prawns	9.50
Peanuts	13.80
Cornflakes	16.00
Rice Krispies	16.00

Vitamin B6 – pyridoxine
Milligrams per 100 g (3.5 oz)

Carrots	0.05
Full-fat milk	0.06
Skimmed milk	0.06
Semi-skimmed milk	0.06
Satsuma	0.07
White bread	0.07
White rice	0.07
Cabbage, boiled	0.08
Cottage cheese	0.08
Cox's apple	0.08
Wholemeal pasta	0.08
Frozen peas	0.08
Spinach, boiled	0.09
Cheddar cheese	0.10
Orange	0.10
Broccoli	0.11
Hovis	0.11
Baked beans	0.12
Boiled egg	0.12
Red kidney beans, cooked	0.12
Wholemeal bread	0.12
Tomatoes	0.14
Almonds	0.15
Cauliflower	0.15

Brussels sprouts	0.19		Shrimps, boiled	1.80
Sweetcorn, boiled	0.21		Parmesan cheese	1.90
Leg of lamb, cooked	0.22		Beef, lean	2.00
Grapefruit juice	0.23		Cod, baked	2.00
Roast chicken	0.26		Cornflakes	2.00
Lentils, boiled	0.28		Pork, cooked	2.00
Banana	0.29		Raw beef mince	2.00
Brazil nuts	0.31		Rice Krispies	2.00
Potatoes, boiled	0.32		Steak, lean, grilled	2.00
Roast turkey	0.33		Edam cheese	2.10
Grilled herring	0.33		Eggs, whole, battery	2.40
Topside of beef, cooked	0.33		Milk, dried, whole	2.40
Avocado	0.36		Milk, dried, skimmed	2.60
Grilled cod	0.38		Eggs, whole, free-range	2.70
Baked salmon	0.57		Kambu seaweed	2.80
Soya flour	0.57		Squid, frozen	2.90
Hazelnuts	0.59		Taramasalata	2.90
Peanuts	0.59		Duck, cooked	3.00
Walnuts	0.67		Turkey, dark meat	3.00
Muesli	1.60		Grapenuts	5.00
Cornflakes	1.80		Tuna in oil	5.00
Rice Krispies	1.80		Herring, cooked	6.00
Special K	2.20		Herring roe, fried	6.00
			Steamed salmon	6.00
Vitamin B12			Bovril	8.30
Micrograms per 100 g (3.5 oz)			Mackerel, fried	10.00
Tempeh	0.10		Rabbit, stewed	10.00
Miso	0.20		Cod's roe, fried	11.00
Quorn	0.30		Pilchards canned in tomato juice	12.00
Full-fat milk	0.40		Oysters, raw	15.00
Skimmed milk	0.40		Nori seaweed	27.50
Semi-skimmed milk	0.40		Sardines in oil	28.00
Marmite	0.50		Lamb's kidney, fried	79.00
Cottage cheese	0.70			
Choux buns	1.00		**Folate/Folic acid**	
Eggs, boiled	1.00		*Micrograms per 100 g (3.5 oz)*	
Eggs, poached	1.00		Cox's apple	4.00
Halibut, steamed	1.00		Leg of lamb, cooked	4.00
Lobster, boiled	1.00		Full-fat milk	6.00
Sponge cake	1.00		Skimmed milk	6.00
Turkey, white meat	1.00		Semi-skimmed milk	6.00
Waffles	1.00		Porridge with semi-skimmed milk	7.00
Cheddar cheese	1.20		Turnip, baked	8.00
Eggs, scrambled	1.20		Sweet potato, boiled	8.00
Squid, fresh	1.30		Cucumber	9.00
Eggs, fried	1.60		Grilled herring	10.00

Roast chicken	10.00		Artichoke	68.00
Avocado	11.00		Hazelnuts	72.00
Grilled cod	12.00		Spinach, boiled	90.00
Banana	14.00		Brussels sprouts	110.00
Roast turkey	15.00		Peanuts	110.00
Carrots	17.00		Muesli	140.00
Sweet potato	17.00		Sweetcorn, boiled	150.00
Tomatoes	17.00		Asparagus	155.00
Topside of beef, cooked	17.00		Chick peas	180.00
Swede, boiled	18.00		Lamb's liver, fried	240.00
Strawberries	20.00		Cornflakes	250.00
Brazil nuts	21.00		Rice Krispies	250.00
Red peppers, raw	21.00		Calves' liver, fried	320.00
Green peppers, raw	23.00			
Rye bread	24.00		**Vitamin C**	
Dates, fresh	25.00		*Milligrams per 100 g (3.5 oz)*	
New potatoes, boiled	25.00		Full-fat milk	1.00
Grapefruit	26.00		Skimmed milk	1.00
Oatcakes	26.00		Semi-skimmed milk	1.00
Cottage cheese	27.00		Red kidney beans	1.00
Baked salmon	29.00		Carrots	2.00
Cabbage, boiled	29.00		Cucumber	2.00
Onions, boiled	29.00		Muesli with dried fruit	2.00
White bread	29.00		Apricots, raw	6.00
Orange	31.00		Avocado	6.00
Baked beans	33.00		Pear	6.00
Cheddar cheese	33.00		Potato, boiled	6.00
Clementines	33.00		Spinach, boiled	8.00
Raspberries	33.00		Cox's apple	9.00
Satsuma	33.00		Turnip	10.00
Blackberries	34.00		Banana	11.00
Rye crispbread	35.00		Frozen peas	12.00
Potato, baked in skin	36.00		Lamb's liver, fried	12.00
Radish	38.00		Pineapple	12.00
Boiled egg	39.00		Dried skimmed milk	13.00
Hovis	39.00		Gooseberries	14.00
Wholemeal bread	39.00		Raw dates	14.00
Red kidney beans, boiled	42.00		Melon	17.00
Potato, baked	44.00		Tomatoes	17.00
Frozen peas	47.00		Cabbage, boiled	20.00
Almonds	48.00		Canteloupe melon	26.00
Parsnips, boiled	48.00		Cauliflower	27.00
Cauliflower	51.00		Satsuma	27.00
Green beans, boiled	57.00		Peach	31.00
Broccoli	64.00		Raspberries	32.00
Walnuts	66.00		Bran flakes	35.00

Grapefruit	36.00
Mangoes	37.00
Nectarine	37.00
Kumquats	39.00
Broccoli	44.00
Lychees	45.00
Unsweetened apple juice	49.00
Orange	54.00
Kiwi fruit	59.00
Brussels sprouts	60.00
Strawberries	77.00
Blackcurrants	115.00

Vitamin D
Micrograms per 100g (3.5 oz)

Skimmed milk	0.01
Whole milk	0.03
Fromage frais	0.05
Cheddar cheese	0.26
Cornflakes	2.80
Rice Krispies	2.80
Kellogg's Start	4.20
Margarine	8.00

Vitamin E
Milligrams per 100 g (3.5 oz)

Semi-skimmed milk	0.03
Boiled potatoes	0.06
Cucumber	0.07
Cottage cheese	0.08
Full-fat milk	0.09
Cabbage, boiled	0.10
Leg of lamb, cooked	0.10
Cauliflower	0.11
Roast chicken	0.11
Frozen peas	0.18
Red kidney beans, cooked	0.20
Wholemeal bread	0.20
Orange	2.4
Topside of beef, cooked	0.26
Banana	0.27
Brown rice, boiled	0.30
Grilled herring	0.30
Lamb's liver, fried	0.32
Baked beans	0.36
Cornflakes	0.40

Pear	0.50
Cheddar cheese	0.53
Carrots	0.56
Lettuce	0.57
Cox's apple	0.59
Grilled cod	0.59
Rice Krispies	0.60
Plums	0.61
Unsweetened orange juice	0.68
Leeks	0.78
Sweetcorn, boiled	0.88
Brussels sprouts	0.90
Broccoli	1.10
Boiled egg	1.11
Tomato	1.22
Watercress	1.46
Parsley	1.70
Spinach, boiled	1.71
Olives	1.99
Butter	2.00
Onions, dried raw	2.69
Mushrooms, fried in corn oil	2.84
Avocado	3.20
Muesli	3.20
Walnuts	3.85
Peanut butter	4.99
Olive oil	5.10
Sweet potato, baked	5.96
Brazil nuts	7.18
Peanuts	10.09
Pine nuts	13.65
Rapeseed oil	18.40
Almonds	23.96
Hazelnuts	24.98
Sunflower oil	48.70

Calcium
Milligrams per 100 g (3.5 oz)

Cox's apple	4.00
Brown rice, boiled	4.00
Potatoes, boiled	5.00
Banana	6.00
Topside of beef, cooked	6.00
White pasta, boiled	7.00
Tomato	7.00
White spaghetti, boiled	7.00

Leg of lamb, cooked	8.00	Green beans	4
Red peppers, raw	8.00	Mushrooms	4
Roast chicken	9.00	Orange	5
Roast turkey	9.00	Lettuce	7
Avocado	11.00	Shrimps	7
Pear	11.00	Carrots	9
Butter	15.00	Banana	10
Cornflakes	15.00	Spinach	10
White rice, boiled	18.00	Scallops	11
Grilled cod	22.00	Butter	13
Lentils, boiled	22.00	Parsnips	13
Baked salmon	29.00	Apple	14
Green peppers, raw	30.00	Hens' eggs	16
Young carrots	30.00	Green (bell) peppers	19
Grilled herring	33.00	Pork chops	20
Wholemeal flour	38.00	Potatoes	24
Turnips, baked	45.00	Fresh chilli	30
Orange	47.00	Rye bread	30
Baked beans	48.00	Lamb chops	42
Wholemeal bread	54.00	Chicken	45
Boiled egg	57.00	Calves' liver	55
Peanuts	60.00	Brewer's yeast	112
Cottage cheese	73.00		
Soya beans, boiled	83.00	**Iron**	
White bread	100.00	*Milligrams per 100 g (3.5 oz)*	
Full-fat milk	115.00	Semi-skimmed milk	0.05
Hovis	120.00	Skimmed milk	0.06
Muesli	120.00	Full-fat milk	0.06
Skimmed milk	120.00	Cottage cheese	0.10
Semi-skimmed milk	120.00	Orange	0.10
Prawns, boiled	150.00	Cox's apple	0.20
Spinach, boiled	150.00	Pear	0.20
Brazil nuts	170.00	White rice	0.20
Yoghurt, low-fat, plain	190.00	Banana	0.30
Soya flour	210.00	Cabbage, boiled	0.30
Almonds	240.00	Cheddar cheese	0.30
White self-raising flour	4.50.00	Avocado	0.40
Sardines	550.00	Grilled cod	0.40
Sprats, fried	710.00	Potatoes, boiled	0.40
Cheddar cheese	720.00	Young carrots, boiled	0.40
Whitebait, fried	860.00	Brown rice, boiled	0.50
		Tomato	0.50
Chromium		White pasta, boiled	0.50
Milligrams per 100 g (3.5 oz)		Baked salmon	0.80
Milk	1	Roast chicken	0.80
Cabbage	4	Roast turkey	0.90

Grilled herring	1.00	Green peppers, raw	24.00
Red peppers, raw	1.00	Roast chicken	24.00
Boiled prawns	1.10	Topside of beef, cooked	24.00
Green peppers, raw	1.20	White bread	24.00
Baked beans	1.40	Avocado	25.00
Wholemeal spaghetti, boiled	1.40	Cheddar cheese	25.00
White bread	1.60	Grilled cod	26.00
Spinach, boiled	1.70	Roast turkey	27.00
Boiled egg	1.90	Leg of lamb, cooked	28.00
White self-raising flour	2.00	Baked salmon	29.00
Brazil nuts	2.50	Baked beans	31.00
Peanuts	2.50	Spinach, boiled	31.00
Leg of lamb, cooked	2.70	Grilled herring	32.00
Wholemeal bread	2.70	Banana	34.00
Topside of beef, cooked	2.80	Lentils, boiled	34.00
Almonds	3.00	Boiled prawns	42.00
Soya beans, boiled	3.00	Wholemeal spaghetti, boiled	42.00
Lentils, boiled	3.50	Brown rice, boiled	43.00
Hovis	3.70	Hovis	56.00
Wholemeal flour	3.90	Soya beans, boiled	63.00
Muesli	5.60	Wholemeal bread	76.00
Cornflakes	6.70	Muesli	85.00
Rice Krispies	6.70	Wholemeal flour	120.00
Soya flour	6.90	Peanuts	210.00
		Soya flour	240.00
		Almonds	270.00
		Brazil nuts	410.00

Magnesium *l = 17*
Milligrams per 100 g (3.5 oz)

Butter	2.00		
Cox's apple	6.00	**Selenium**	
Turnip, baked	6.00	*Micrograms per 100 g (3.5 oz)*	
Young carrots	6.00	Full-fat milk	1.00
Tomato	7.00	Semi-skimmed milk	1.00
Cottage cheese	9.00	Skimmed milk	1.00
Orange	10.00	Baked beans	2.00
Full-fat milk	11.00	Cornflakes	2.00
White rice, boiled	11.00	Orange	2.00
Semi-skimmed milk	11.00	Peanuts	3.00
Skimmed milk	12.00	Almonds	4.00
Boiled egg	12.00	Cottage cheese	4.00
Cornflakes	14.00	White rice	4.00
Potatoes, boiled	14.00	White self-raising flour	4.00
Red peppers, raw	14.00	Soya beans, boiled	5.00
White pasta	15.00	Boiled egg	11.00
White spaghetti, boiled	15.00	Cheddar cheese	12.00
White self-raising flour	20.00	White bread	28.00

Wholemeal bread	35.00
Lentils, boiled	40.00
Wholemeal flour	53.00

Zinc

Milligrams per 100 g (3.5 oz)

Butter	0.10
Pear	0.10
Orange	0.10
Red peppers, raw	0.10
Banana	0.20
Young carrots	0.20
Cornflakes	0.30
Potatoes, boiled	0.30
Avocado	0.40
Full-fat milk	0.40
Skimmed milk	0.40
Green peppers, raw	0.40
Semi-skimmed milk	0.40
Baked beans	0.50
Grilled cod	0.50
Grilled herring	0.50
White pasta	0.50
Tomatoes	0.50
Cottage cheese	0.60
Spinach, boiled	0.60
White bread	0.60
White self-raising flour	0.60
Brown rice	0.70
White rice	0.70
Soya beans, boiled	0.90
Wholemeal spaghetti, boiled	1.10
Boiled egg	1.30
Lentils, boiled	1.40
Roast chicken	1.50
Boiled prawns	1.60

Wholemeal bread	1.80
Hovis	2.10
Cheddar cheese	2.30
Roast turkey	2.40
Muesli	2.50
Wholemeal flour	2.90
Almonds	3.20
Peanuts	3.50
Brazil nuts	4.20
Leg of lamb, cooked	5.30
Topside of beef, cooked	5.50

Essential fatty acids

Exact amounts of these fats are hard to quantify. Good sources for the two families of essential fatty acids are given.

Omega-6 series essential fatty acids

Sunflower oil
Rapeseed oil
Corn oil
Almonds
Walnuts
Brazil nuts
Sunflower seeds
Soya products including tofu

Omega-3 series essential fatty acids

Mackerel ⎫
Herring ⎬ fresh cooked or smoked/pickled
Salmon ⎭

Walnuts and walnut oil
Rapeseed oil
Soya products and soya bean oil

INDEX

For nutritional content of foods see pages 275–82